MEDICAL STATISTICS ON PERSONAL COMPUTERS

A guide to the appropriate use of statistical packages

SECOND EDITION

MEDICAL STATISTICS ON PERSONAL COMPUTERS

A guide to the appropriate use of statistical packages

SECOND EDITION

R A Brown
Department of Mathematics and Computer Science,
University of Dundee
and
J Swanson Beck
Department of Pathology
Ninewells Hospital and Medical School,
Dundee

©BMJ Publishing Group 1990, 1994

First edition 1990
Second edition 1994

British Library Cataloguing in Publication Data

A catalogue record for this book is available from the British Library.

ISBN 0 7279 0771 9

Typeset, printed and bound in Great Britain by
Latimer Trend & Co Ltd, Plymouth, England

Contents

Foreword to second edition

In the relatively short time since the first edition appeared personal computer systems have become more powerful, and most statistical packages have increased the range of calculations they can perform and have improved the attractiveness of their "look and feel" on screen. However, they have not become more intelligent. The onus is still on the user to choose an appropriate statistical analysis, so that informed understanding of the use of statistical techniques is still of great importance. The book has been extended by the inclusion of material on survival analysis, statistical power calculations, notes on some of the more popular packages, and advice on the best way to write up statistical analyses in medical papers. The authors have also corrected a number of errors in the original text, some of which were kindly pointed out by readers of the first edition.

R A Brown, J Swanson Beck
November 1993

Introduction

Recent developments in microcomputer technology, particularly the introduction of the IBM personal computer and the mass production of inexpensive "clones," have put within reach of the budgets of most laboratories relatively powerful machines such as the XT and AT models. In response to growing demand computer software has been written to perform a wide range of tasks, and very sophisticated programs are now available at modest prices. Consequently, most workers in pathology laboratories are likely to have access to computer power that could not have been imagined a decade ago. As a result the users of statistical techniques need no longer be concerned with the arithmetical and algebraic details of various statistical methods and can concentrate instead on understanding the underlying ideas and basic principles of statistical analysis.

This book has been written to show how personal computers can be used to facilitate the analysis of data. It is our intention:

(i) to explain the rational basis of widely applicable statistical methods without requiring the reader to understand the underlying algebra; and

(ii) to summarise the limitations of the various statistical procedures so that the user can make an informed choice when analysing data.

We do not intent to present an extensive account of the design of clinical trials as the techniques and approaches applicable to this type of work have recently been discussed fairly exhaustively.[1 2] We shall concentrate, instead, on statistical methods applicable to most laboratory investigations. Details of the algebraic formulae used for particular statistical methods may be obtained from standard texts.[3-5]

1

Data handling

Organisation of information in the personal computer

In certain specialised applications data are transferred directly from analytical apparatus to a personal computer via a connecting cable. Diverse observations made on each individual patient or specimen, however, will more commonly be keyed in manually before any statistical analysis can be done. The computer can store data in files on a floppy or hard disc, depending on the configuration of the machine. The way in which files are stored need not concern us here as the disc operating system (DOS) takes care of this.

To put the data into the file system the user has three options: the data can be entered by using (a) a proprietary Spreadsheet program, (b) a proprietary Database Management System (DBMS), or (c) the data entry facilities within the statistical analysis package.

Spreadsheets were invented in the 1970s to assist business people in making financial calculations, but they were very quickly adopted in areas of application which had nothing to do with finance. In financial calculations you usually have several columns of figures— for example, unit prices and quantities of goods ordered—and you want to make up an invoice, say, which involves calculating the actual price for each invoiced item by multiplying quantity ordered by unit price. These figures will need to be placed in a third column. If value added tax (or local sales tax) has to be added then a further calculation is required, the values in the actual price column must be multiplied by the appropriate tax rate, and the results must be placed in a fourth column. The price charged will be the sum of these two columns and this will need to be displayed as a fifth column. Finally, these columns must be added up to give the total price excluding tax, the total tax, and the total price including tax.

Anyone who has struggled with the data resulting from a biomedical investigation will recognise that the types of calculation involved in preparing an invoice, adding columns together, taking a percentage of each value in a column and so on, are familiar operations. Hence the widespread adoption of spreadsheets as aids to data manipulation outside the financial world. There are several professionally produced spreadsheet programs on the market, any computer magazine will list perhaps a dozen or more. One of the market leaders is called Lotus 1-2-3, others are Supercalc and VP Planner, but Lotus 1-2-3 has more or less set the standard in this field and has sold over twenty million copies. All spreadsheets work in essentially the same way, but the user must check that the spreadsheet they have chosen stores data on file in a manner compatible with the statistical package they intend to use.

Spreadsheet programs are incredibly easy to use. Initially the user is presented with a blank screen organised into columns. Each row can therefore represent a subject and each column the value of a particular type of observation. Data may be typed from the computer keyboard into any row or column. There is also a special facility for defining the values which are to go into a particular column in terms of the values present in other columns. For instance, you might wish to give an instruction such as "make each value in column 3 equal to the corresponding value in column 1 minus the corresponding value in column 2." Once such an instruction has been given the spreadsheet program will automatically calculate these values, and what is more it will store this definition as part of the spreadsheet data file. This means that if the user subsequently changes any of the values in columns 1 or 2 the corresponding changes to column 3 will occur automatically. This is an example of the use of a very simple arithmetic expression, but all sorts of much more complicated column definitions are available; you could, if you wished, define column 5 in a particular spreadsheet as the logarithm of the squares of the values in columns 1 and 2 divided by the square root of the ratio of the values in columns 3 and 4.

There are also special commands for entering repetitive values into a column. For example, data may be gathered on 300 subjects, of whom 120 are healthy controls, 105 are patients with pulmonary tuberculosis and 75 are patients with leprosy. To distinguish the three groups it is customary to use codes such as 1 = normal, 2 = pulmonary tuberculosis, and 3 = leprosy, so that one variable in the data file should consist of 120 ones, followed by 105 twos, and then 75 threes. The spreadsheet program has special facilities for defining a column consisting of 120 ones, 105 twos, and 75 threes in that order, so that the user is relieved of the drudgery of typing in all this repetitive information.

Databases The spreadsheet can be seen as the electronic equivalent of a large table. An alternative manual system of record keeping is to have a record card for each individual with labelled spaces for the data. This results in a stack of record cards rather than a table: the computer implementation of this is a DBMS. The user designs a master form which contains blank spaces for the data and this is stored on disc. To facilitate data entry it is a good idea to make the screen format look like the corresponding manual record card. To store a series of records the DBMS presents the user with a fresh pro-forma on screen for each record: each item can then be inserted into the appropriate blank space. This method is preferable when a large number of records have to be filed; the use of the master as a prompt to the user greatly reduces the incidence of errors.

Good statistical packages have data entry facilities which usually operate on something like the spreadsheet principle so it is not essential to use one of the spreadsheet or DBMS programs, but many workers find such programs convenient. It must be emphasised, however, that individual data management systems may store data on disc in different formats. If a proprietary program is used then care must be taken to ensure that the format is compatible with that of the statistical package.

The method is very simple in Statgraphics. The first procedure in transferring a file from a spreadsheet in Lotus 1-2-3 is to introduce a temporary change to the "System Profile" to ensure that the import pathway is switched to the appropriate Lotus file on the hard disc. The "Import" menu is then called up, import file type is given as Lotus, the original ".WKS" file name is entered and the new Statgraphics file name specified; after pressing the "F6" key the transfer will be accomplished automatically.

Variability

If there were no variability in results there would not be any need for statistical analysis to aid in the interpretation of data from experiments or clinical observations. We all appreciate that variability in our results is often great and we optimistically resort to

3

statistical analysis for support or guidance. There is no single cause of variability, which can arise from three main sources.

(1) Methodology All methods of measurement give results that are estimates of the underlying absolute value. Those which are based on direct physical measurement, such as length, weight, or temperature, are usually relatively accurate, provided the apparatus is functioning properly and no errors are introduced in recording, but it is clear that the more indirect the measurement process the greater the variability that will arise. When a metabolic activity is assessed by use of a radioactive tracer, the counts that result will be subject to Poisson variability arising from the intermittent process of atomic disintegration. Even greater variability may arise if some form of interpolation or mathematical modelling is required to interpret the experimental results. An important distinction must be remembered: *accuracy* is an indication of how close the measurement will be to the absolute value; *precision* is a measure of how close replicates will be to each other. High precision will arise from good technical work, but it does not necessarily indicate good accuracy. Precision can, in principle, be measured quite easily as all that has to be done is to compare a series of replicate measurements. Accuracy is much more difficult to ascertain as the replicate measurements of a known standard must be compared. This standard has to be specially prepared and you must be sure that its value is actually known and that it does not deteriorate with time.

(2) Sampling Because it is not usually practicable to measure all the material in a specimen and it is certainly not possible to measure all relevant aspects of a patient, there will inevitably be variability inherent in the actual part of the sample that is being analysed. Sometimes this will not be great—for example, one aliquot from a serum sample is unlikely to differ widely from another, provided deterioration has not occurred in the intervening time—but whenever tissue samples, cells, or particles are involved there is considerable potential for variation among samples (even serial histological sections can vary considerably from each other), and greater differences may be seen between different biopsy specimens when the underlying disease is focal.

(3) Human variation Even in healthy subjects there can be variation, reflecting different genetic backgrounds or biological

4

experience. Moreover, there can be variations with time due to oscillations of physiological behaviour that may or may not be in phase with an easily recognisable periodicity, such as diurnal rhythm. There are even greater sources of variation in patients in whom severity of disease or response to treatment differs.

In the planning of any investigation it is essential that care is taken to minimise controllable sources of variability and to recognise the aspects that are beyond the control of the investigator. In this way the investigator optimises the chance of getting data which can be analysed successfully. It must always be remembered that the basic purpose of an investigation is not to accumulate numbers and to be busy, but rather to draw conclusions from a particular study that can legitimately be applied throughout the world to improve understanding of biomedical mechanisms, or the natural history of disease, and to provide the basis for better treatment of patients in clinical practice. It is important, however, to process enough data to enable statistically sound conclusions to be drawn.

Types of investigation

Statisticians distinguish between experimental investigations and observational studies, and the distinction is important as there are more problems with the interpretation of the results of a statistical analysis applied to the latter. *Experimental investigations* aim to compare two or more *treatments*, such as the administration of various drugs, applied to groups of subjects, or to investigate the consequences of deliberate variation of *factors* which are controlled by the investigator. A typical example of a study of this type would be the investigation of the effect of storage temperature on the recovery of bone marrow cells for transplantation. The sample of bone marrow was split into aliquots each of which was stored at one of a number of predetermined temperatures, and the viability of the cells was measured at the end of the fixed in vitro storage periods. The aliquots to be stored at each temperature were chosen at random, and identical methods were used to measure viability in all samples so that the effect of other variables was minimised.

In an experimental investigation the investigator has complete freedom to decide which experimental subject should be assigned to each treatment. There will inevitably be unsuspected differences between people even within a homogeneous group, and to

5

ensure that these are evened out and so do not bias observed mean responses it is essential to allocate patients randomly to the treatment groups. This process is known as *randomisation* and it ensures the validity of the inference that observed differences between groups are caused by the different treatment they have received.

In summary, an experimental investigation entails the following:

(i) *replication*, several patients or units of experimental material allocated to each group;

(ii) allocation of subjects to treatments under the control of the investigator;

(iii) randomisation.

In contrast, an *observational study* usually lacks the second and third elements listed above. For example, an observational study of the prognostic value of microscopical and other features of primary tumours in breast cancer might proceed by extracting all available case records and specimens. Measurements or gradings of potentially important characteristics, such as tumour size, and of other possible prognostic indicators, such as the extent of lymph node disease, would be recorded. The investigator might then divide the cases into two groups—poor and good survival—and look for some subset of the recorded features, a discriminating subset, which differs substantially between the two groups. Once this has been found, one can combine the value of several features in the discriminating subset to yield a score for each patient, and this is used as a predictor of survival in new cases. Note that the composition of the groups is not, and cannot be, controlled by the investigator as it is clearly impossible to allocate patients randomly to the poor and good survival groups. Consequently, considerable caution must be exercised in ascribing the observed differences among the prognostic features to the overt difference between survival experience. There could well be some unsuspected factors which were seriously unbalanced between the two groups that could equally well be the explanation of the observed differences. It is therefore essential to verify the results of potentially important observational studies by the accumulation of further data in follow up studies in which the discriminating criteria are applied to new cases.

Statistical packages for personal computers

There are several good quality statistical packages available which, when used in a knowledgeable way, allow the experimenter to use many more methods than is practical using traditional paper calculations. This book will be illustrated by reference to the working of two well known packages—Minitab and Statgraphics. These packages have a good reputation in the field of statistics and have been evaluated by bodies such as the American Statistical Association, which runs a continuing programme of package review and evaluation. Both have clearly written, unambiguous manuals. There are other less expensive packages but we have not used them; the principles that we explain in this book should be generally applicable.

The data can be entered directly into the statistical package from the keyboard, or indirectly from a spreadsheet or a database. Statgraphics uses a spreadsheet format for the entry of data. Data are stored as variables, each occupying a column, and these variables are in turn organised into files. The files are stored on the hard disc. Each variable has to be given a name by the user, the naming convention is quite flexible, up to 10 alpha numeric characters may be used to make up a variable name, the only restriction being that the name must begin with a letter. Thus "age", "scx", "wbc", and "OKT4" are all valid names but "3-HTdR" is not as it begins with a numeral and contains a hyphen. Each file must also be given a name by the user with a similar flexibility in the naming convention, up to eight alpha numeric characters are allowed, beginning with a letter. Hence "lymphoma", "Crohns", and "Hodgkins" are valid file names but "Crohn's" is not as it contains an apostrophe.

To make it easy to see what is stored on the hard disc Statgraphics creates a "data directory" at the start of each session. This is a complete list of all the Statgraphics data files and the variables stored in them. By moving a cursor to any desired variable it is possible to display its contents, get a printed copy of it, or insert it as the name of a variable within a Statgraphics procedure.

To create a new file containing several variables you select the "Data Management" option from the main menu. After selection of the relevant options from two submenus you are faced with a spreadsheet display into which you can insert the names of variables (as column headings) and enter the values of these variables from the keyboard. This is done using the Statgraphics "full screen editor," a subprogram designed to make data entry or editing of Statgraphics data files particularly easy. Once the file is complete, or indeed at any intermediate stage, it can be saved on to disc. If a file is particularly long the user may wish to create it over several Statgraphics sessions, adding further data to the file at each session.

Thereafter the statistical package is driven by the operator selecting a procedure from a menu (fig 1.1) or by a system of brief but memorable commands, whichever is appropriate to the design of the package or the convenience of the user. At various points in certain analyses, the user is allowed to select from a range of options to see plots or perform supplementary analyses. All of the common methods of display, summary, and analysis are literally at the user's fingertips, but current statistical packages, being essentially "unintelligent," are incapable of advising on the most appropriate method for a particular data set and this remains the prerogative of the user.

STATGRAPHICS *statistical graphics system*

DATA MANAGEMENT AND SYSTEM UTILITIES	*TIME SERIES PROCEDURES*
A Data management	L Forecasting
B System environment	M Quality control
C Report writer and graphics replay	N Smoothing
D Plotter interface	O Time series analysis

PLOTTING AND DESCRIPTIVE STATISTICS	*ADVANCED PROCEDURES*
E Plotting functions	
F Descriptive methods	P Categorical data analysis
G Estimation and testing	Q Multivariate methods
H Distribution functions	R Nonparametric methods
I Exploratory data analysis	S Sampling
	T Experimental design

ANOVA AND REGRESSION ANALYSIS	*MATHEMATICAL AND USER PROCEDURES*
J Analysis of variance	U Mathematical functions
K Regression analysis	V Supplementary operations

Use cursor keys to highlight desired section. Then press ENTER.

Figure 1.1   The Statgraphics main menu allows the user to choose from a wide range of options.

The statistical packages arrange the data in spreadsheet form so it is important to identify variables unambiguously and to identify missing values. The conventions of the package must be rigidly adhered to if malfunction is to be avoided.

Types of data

Data obtained by observation or measurement in the laboratory or clinic can be of three different types which must be distinguished clearly as different methods of analysis are appropriate for the various types of data.

Nominal data—the observations are classified into categories that are different in character and cannot be measured or ordered—for example, hair colour or race—often the named character can be only present $(+)$ or absent $(-)$.

Ordinal data—here the observations refer to a common character and they can be grouped into a limited number of categories which can be ordered in an ascending series or rank, such as staging of cancer: commonly such data are presented as $+$, $++$, or $+++$, but numbers can also be used to describe the categories so that there is a danger of confusion of this form of ranking with true measurements. It is essential to remember that in ordinal data the grouping is only semiquantitative and that $+$ is not half as big as $++$: moreover, the intervals between successive categories will probably be different.

Continuous data—is the term used to describe observations made on a scale which has a natural zero and a well defined unit of measurement, such as length: the observations will usually be expressed as decimal numbers.

Both nominal and ordinal data give rise to counts of the frequency of occurrence of the various categories within the groups of subjects under investigation and these counts are naturally whole numbers. They may be converted into rates, proportions, or percentages; when expressed in this form they appear to be decimal numbers but they are essentially different in character from continuous data and need appropriately different statistical treatment.

9

Appendix

Missing values

If certain observations are not available then this must be indicated during data entry by using a "missing value code" to represent them. In Statgraphics a missing value is indicated by leaving a blank in the corresponding position in the worksheet; in Minitab an asterisk is used instead of a blank.

When the experimenter is aware that there are missing data the manual for the package should be consulted to verify if there is some method of specifying missing values, otherwise every analysis will have to be preceded by a data editing session to weed out the cases with missing values—a very tedious business.

Importing spreadsheet and database files

Importing is the name given to the process for transferring data files from proprietary spreadsheets and DBMS into a statistical package. Statgraphics will cope with files from Lotus 1-2-3, Symphony, and dBase III. Minitab can read files from Lotus 1-2-3 only, but certain "Lotus-clones" may be acceptable.

Command lines

The Minitab package uses commands in preference to a menu system; the user specifies the task to be done by typing a command line. Minitab uses command lines which are reasonably memorable—for example, the sequence of commands:

```
NAME C1 'height'
NAME C2 'weight'
DOTPLOT 'height'
PLOT 'height' vs 'weight'
```

names the first and second columns of the worksheet height and weight and produces a dotplot of height and a plot of height against weight.

2

Summarising data.

Data displays and statistical summaries

It is important that any conclusion to be drawn from an experiment is intuitively acceptable as "common sense" and that statistical methods are used to facilitate objective assessment of results. It is therefore essential that the experimenter examines the "raw" data from every experiment. Graphical displays have an immediate visual impact and a compactness that is always absent from numerical tables. Differences between groups, variability within groups, time trends, or other forms of associations between sets of measurements can be investigated and communicated by simple well designed graphical displays. Such displays are a valuable feature of all good statistical packages—Statgraphics is particularly good in this respect. There are no rigid rules for the selection of the most appropriate method of display to show the magnitude and variability of the observations in any particular experiment. The choice is guided by informed common sense, but the chosen format should, in the first instance, present all the original observations (not just condensed summaries) to allow the observer to "eyeball" the results and judge the plausibility of any conclusions presented.

A basic assumption of several widely used statistical methods is that the groups of results being compared have similar variability and this can often be assessed by visual inspection of their distributions. Such preliminary examination of the data can usually be performed conveniently on the visual display screen of the microcomputer. When the data sets are large some summarised form of display may be needed because of the confusion of overlapping points on the screen, but, whatever the method, it must present a fair and unbiased view of the variability of the data.

The dot plot—All the observations are displayed by symbols in a vertical array alongside an appropriate scale (fig 2.1A). This plot gives a visual indication of the magnitude and spread of each set of values, but comparisons of sets of values are more difficult than they appear: it is therefore useful to supplement the display with indicators of the group means at least.

The histogram is an alternative display that is useful when each group consists of a large number of measurements (100 or more). The interval of the measurement scale which contains all the data is divided into equal subintervals and the number of values falling into each subinterval is represented by a rectangle with height proportional to this number. Care is needed in the selection of the subintervals as too many will reduce the number of values in each one, emphasising minor fluctuation, and too few will obscure the true variability of the data. The Statgraphics package is capable of generating histogram displays automatically but the user can easily choose a preferred style that overrides the inbuilt criteria for selection of interval size.

The fact that the individual observations are not shown and that the number of intervals is chosen subjectively makes this a poor choice for final presentation of results. Because of this, many scientific journals have a policy of not publishing data in histogram format.

Summary statistics to indicate location, spread, and symmetry

There are a few simple statistics that can convey a lot of information about a set of observations. Most standard statistical methods for analysing two or more sets of measurements assume that:

(i) each set has more or less the same variability;

(ii) the distribution of values around the mean is more or less symmetrical (for "parametric" analyses), or has a similar shape in each group;

(iii) there are no outliers (values far removed from the main body) in the data.

Magnitude An indication of the "middle" of the data gives useful information when attempting to determine whether groups of data are similar or different. Two statistics commonly used for this purpose are the *mean* (arithmetical average) and the *median* (middle value when the observations are ranked in order). Either value will be equally informative when the distribution is symmetrical but the mean forms the basis of certain standard methods

12

for assessing differences between groups. If the mean and the median are quite different this indicates serious asymmetry, and methods of statistical analysis based on medians and on rank order of data will be necessary (details are given in later chapters of this book). Outliers do not affect the median but they may make the mean unrepresentative.

Spread—Again there is a choice of summary statistics. The *standard deviation* (SD) is widely used, but it is valid only when the data are more or less symmetrical: it is the square root of the average of the squared deviations of the data values from the mean. An alternative is the *interquartile range* (fig 2.1B): when the data are ordered the upper and lower quartiles are the values that separate off the upper and lower 25% of the values; thus the interquartile range measures the middle 50% of the data and this is valid whether or not the data are symmetrically distributed. The *range*— the difference between the largest and smallest values—is much less informative because it is so sensitive to outliers. All these summary statistics are readily generated in microcomputer packages.

Symmetry This can be assessed from a "box and whisker plot" which indicates graphically the median, quartiles, and range of a

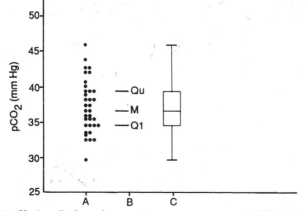

Figure 2.1   Various displays of transcutaneous measurements of pCO$_2$ in forearm skin of normal subjects. (A) A dot plot of the data. (B) The interquartile range spans in central 50% of the data. (C) The box whisker plot suppresses details but indicates spread and symmetry.

13

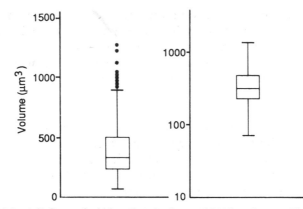

Figure 2.2 (A) Box and whisker plot of volumes of 300 lymphocytes. The distribution is noticeably asymmetrical: in this situation the package calculates the length of the upper whisker as one and a half times the interquartile range (length of rectangle) and the outlying points are plotted individually (see text). (B) Box and whisker plot of the logarithms of the same data: the transformation has made the distribution symmetrical.

set of data and can easily be generated in both packages (fig 2.1C). The central 50% of the data is represented by a rectangle extending from the lower to the upper quartile, the median being indicated by a bar across the rectangle. The "whiskers" extend to the extremes unless there are values which are far away from the central 50% (outliers), in which case the length of the corresponding whisker is set at one and a half times the interquartile range, and the outlying points are plotted individually.

Sometimes asymmetrical data sets can be converted into a more or less symmetrical form by *"transformation"* of the raw results by taking logarithms, square roots, or other simple mathematical functions (fig 2.2), and such procedures can be performed automatically with most packages. Care should be taken if any values are less than zero because logarithms or square roots of negative numbers do not exist. Most packages will insert a "missing value code" in place of an impossible value when transforming; care should be taken to ascertain that the data are not unwittingly corrupted. A useful device is to add a suitable number to all observations to remove negative numbers. Transformation of data is a useful approach; if it is successful it permits the use of statistical methods which require symmetrical distributions on data that are clearly asymmetrical in their raw form. Care is of course necessary when interpreting analyses performed on transformed data; in particular, it is necessary to "back transform" the values resulting from statistical analysis—for example, mean, confidence intervals, etc—before attempting a biological or clinical interpretation of the outcome of the analysis.

Displays to be avoided

One of the commonest forms of data presentation seen in articles published in biomedical journals is the "mean and error bar" plot. Here the original data are not shown, but the mean of each set is plotted with two equal bars above and below (fig 2.3). This type of plot has little to recommend it: it is misleading in several ways.

Firstly, the number of observations in each category is not clearly apparent and so disparity between size of groups being compared or the presence of a very small group that may not be representative can be obscured.

Secondly, the presentation of the equal sized error bars above and below the mean can imply that the data are symmetrically distributed, but the reader cannot assess this for him/herself.

Thirdly, the basis of the calculation of the length of the error bars may be misleading because the indicated range will contain only about 70% of the observations if the standard deviation is chosen. Choice of the standard error of the mean (SEM)—SD divided by square root of number of observations—to indicate

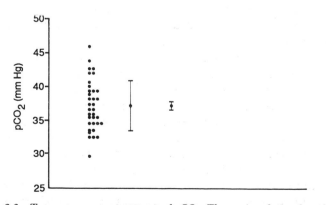

Figure 2.3 Transcutaneous measurement of pCO_2. The mean and error bar plot (larger bars) understates the variability: using the SEM (smaller bars) gives a very misleading impression of variability.

variability is even more misleading as the real extent of variability will be seriously understated, particularly for large samples.

It is clearly not very sensible to replace sets of two or three observations by their mean and standard deviation as the actual values could just as easily be presented and would more clearly tell the story.

Outliers

Occasional values that are considerably larger or smaller than the main group are termed *outliers*. Such observations are commoner than is popularly supposed, but they are unlikely to be appreciated unless the data are displayed using either a dot or box and whisker plot format. Sometimes an outlier is an artefact due to an error in transcription or instrument reading, sometimes it has resulted from inclusion of a result that is inappropriate—for example, erroneous selection of a patient or misclassification of an observation. It is good practice to check the validity of outlier observations, but each observation must be accepted unless there is clear evidence that it is artefactual.

Most of the standard methods that use means and standard deviations are adversely affected by the presence of outliers. Methods which use medians, quartiles, and ranks are generally much less vulnerable to distortion by outliers. It is not possible to give guidelines on how to deal with outliers. Perhaps the safest policy is to be constantly aware of the potential hazards and when outliers are encountered to analyse the data with and without the inclusion of the suspect values. When the results remain substantially unchanged, then you can be reassured that the conclusions drawn from the statistical analysis have not been unduly influenced by the outlier values. When the analyses disagree, however, it is obvious that the outlier values are influencing the analysis. In this situation advice should be sought from a professional statistician who may advise the use of a more valid method of analysis with statistical procedures that are less influenced by outliers.

The normal distribution

Many standard statistical analyses of continuous data are based on the assumption that the spread of values across the population can be described by the so-called "normal" distribution. This form of distribution was originally selected as the basis of much statistical work because it is unimodal and symmetrical, with a high proportion of values relatively close to the mean and decreasing concentration of values in the "tails" of the distribution, similar to many distributions observed in practice. It is undoubtedly a convenient approximation for many sets of data, but it would be wrong to assume that this particular distribution was a biologically "natural" pattern to which all "good" data conform—for example, the distribution of survival times of patients with cancer is not well approximated by the normal distribution.

The normal distribution curve illustrates the way in which a measurement might be expected to vary across a population (fig 2.4) The peak of the curve is located at the population mean and there is a precise relation between the population mean and standard deviation and the proportion of measurements lying within any specified range. For example, the statement that 95% of the values will be within 1·96 population standard deviations either side of the population mean is true for every normal distribution.

As normality is an important assumption for several statistical methods it is important to be able to assess whether a particular set of data shows evidence of serious non-normality. The common methods of statistical analysis are fairly "robust to non-normality" provided that:

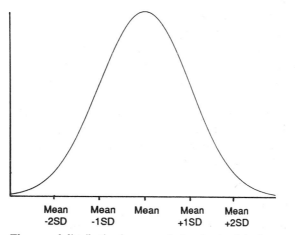

Mean Mean Mean Mean Mean
-2SD -1SD   +1SD +2SD

Figure 2.4   The normal distribution is symmetrical and unimodal: the area under any portion of the curve indicates the probability that an observation will lie within the corresponding range—for example, 68% of observation will lie within 1 SD of the mean.

(i) the data are more or less symmetrically distributed;

(ii) the spread of results is similar in the groups being compared;

(iii) there are no outliers in the data.

Such methods can give rise to misleading results if these requirements are not met.

A simple graphical technique known as normal plotting may be used to assess normality. When performed manually the data values in a single sample are ordered and each value is plotted against the value you would expect to observe if the data were normally distributed. If the data are approximately normally distributed then the plotted points should show a straight line trend. The method is tedious to use manually but with suitable programs a normal plot can be displayed within minutes on a microcomputer. In Statgraphics the individual observations are displayed on an appropriate scale and the best fitting straight line is included so that visual assessment of departure from linearity can be made. If the data are effectively normally distributed the plotted points will be close to the fitted line, but will show pronounced deviations when the data are seriously non-normal.

To indicate how the method works in practice, consider the data on survival times of a group of patients with breast cancer,

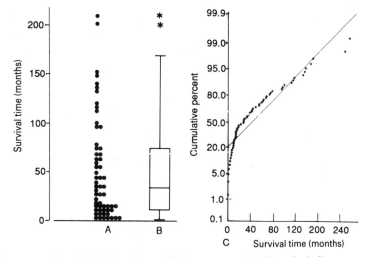

Figure 2.5 Survival of 60 patients with breast cancer (A) Dot plot indicates asymmetry; (B) box and whisker plot indicates that the upper 50% of the survival times are spread over a much greater range than the lower 50%; (C) normal plot shows pronounced curvature, hence the data distribution is very non-normal.

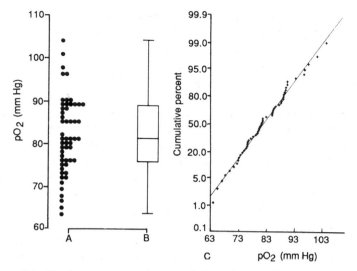

Figure 2.6   Transcutaneous measurements of pO₂ in forearm skin of 54 normal subjects. (A) Dot plot shows no pronounced asymmetry; (B) box and whisker plot clearly indicates near symmetry of the distribution; the median is more or less centrally placed, the whiskers are of almost equal length; (C) normal plot   no serious departure from normality.

displayed as a dot plot in fig 2.5A, a box and whisker plot in fig 2.5B, and as a normal plot in fig 2.5C. Mean survival at 58·5 months is small compared with the sample standard deviation (45 months), which indicates possible asymmetry. The box and whisker plot confirms this, indicating serious asymmetry, and the normal plot, which shows considerable curvature, rules out the normal distribution as an adequate approximation to these data. For comparison, fig 2.6 shows the corresponding displays for a set of 60 normally distributed measurements (in this case the pO₂ in the normal forearm skin measured transcutaneously): the pattern of points shows no serious departure from the fitted line.

19

3

Analysis of data from one or two groups: confidence intervals and significance tests

Populations and samples

The previous chapter described methods for displaying and summarising data. Usually this is not an end in itself, and research workers will wish to extend their conclusions from their samples or experiments to medical practice in general by statistical analysis. It is an essential precondition of valid statistical inference that the groups of subjects included in an investigation are selected randomly from the populations which are being compared, and its aim is to make statements about these global populations based on sample data.

One of the simplest forms of investigation is the comparison of measurements made on two well defined groups of individuals which differ in some clearly specified way—for example, medical treatment, pathological state. The subjects in each group must constitute a random sample from the corresponding population, and as far as practicable, the only major difference between the two groups should be the factor under investigation.

Before the start of an investigation it is essential to define clearly the populations to be sampled when the investigation is expected to result in recommendations of methods of treatment, diagnosis, or prognosis. Failing this, although it is still possible to carry through all stages of a statistical analysis, the final conclusions will be less valuable because they will refer to poorly defined populations. It is regrettable that many scientific reports of otherwise clearly described investigations lack unambiguous definition of criteria for group selection.

An entire population may be accessible at the time of data collection but cost precludes the measurement of every subject. In other situations, especially in disease of gradual onset, the observer can identify fully established disease, but even though he or she is aware of their presence he or she does not have the access or aptitude to identify subjects with presymptomatic defects, such as Alzheimer's disease. In either situation the investigator will make measurements on groups of individuals who have been selected randomly from the corresponding populations. Consequently, there must always be some uncertainty in any general conclusions concerning differences between the populations inferred from differences between the samples, and so the methods used to summarise the conclusions must be based on probability.

The kind of general statements which may be validly made often refer to population means, so it is essential to have a clear idea of what a population mean is and the use to which it can be put. For any specified measurement which could be made on every individual in a well defined population, the population mean is just the value which would be obtained if each member of the population were measured and the mean of all the measurements was calculated. Because biomedical investigations invariably rely on samples to provide information it is clear that a population mean is something that can never be determined. Instead, you must rely on the information provided by the sample mean. As long as the sample is randomly selected from the population you may use the sample mean to estimate the population mean. The use of the word "estimate" serves to indicate that the sample mean cannot provide complete knowledge of the population mean, there will always be some uncertainty about the exact population mean value. How much uncertainty there will be depends on the size of the sample, in general large samples allow a population mean to be estimated more precisely than small ones.

Fortunately, it is never necessary to know the exact value of a population mean; a reasonably precise estimate will always suffice. For example, although it might be fairly interesting to know that the use of a particular technique would increase the yield of viable cells by 47·398% (population mean), an investigator would be quite satisfied with the information that the technique was likely to increase yield by between 45% and 50%, which is the kind of

21

information we can expect to obtain from an investigation based on random sampling. If a closer estimate is required then the investigator merely has to increase the sample size.

If every individual in a population were to be measured we would usually be aware of considerable variation among the measured values. The population standard deviation, which is just the standard deviation of all the values, would be one way of quantifying this variability. This is another quantity which we can never know in practice, but it is important to be able to estimate it.

For example, whether a particular diagnostic test will be useful for screening purposes will depend on the overlap between the values obtained for normal healthy members of the population and those who require treatment. Implicit in this is the idea of two populations, which may be referred to as the healthy population and the abnormal population. The extent of overlap of the distribution of measurements in the two populations depends both on the difference between the population means and on the relative sizes of the population standard deviations.

This is illustrated in fig 3.1 where the bell-shaped curves are meant to indicate the population distributions of the test results. The position of the peak of a curve indicates the population mean, and its breadth is related to the population standard deviation. Consider the vertical line in fig 3.1A, corresponding to a test result of 130 units. The area under the curve labelled "healthy" to the right of this line indicates the proportion of the healthy population who will have a test result above 130 units. In the same way the area under the curve labelled "abnormal" to the left of the vertical line indicates the proportion of abnormal subjects who will have a test result below 130 units. Both proportions are quite large, each being of the order of 30–40%. If the rather naive decision rule, "classify as healthy if the test result is 130 units or less and as abnormal if it is more than 130 units" is used, then it is quite clear that the rule is not going to perform very well. In the long run 30–40% of healthy subjects will be misclassified as abnormal and a similar proportion of abnormal subjects will be misclassified as healthy. By moving the decision point up the scale it is possible to reduce the proportion of healthy subjects who would be misclassified, but only at the cost of misclassifying more abnormal subjects.

There is no good solution in this situation; the population means are too close together and the population standard deviations are too large for there to be any prospect of obtaining a decision rule

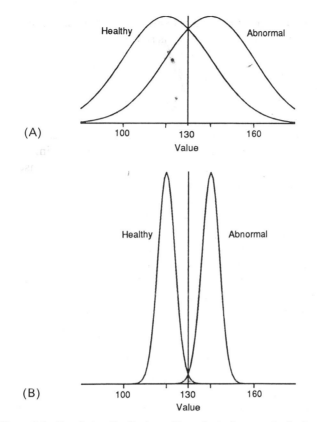

Figure 3.1 Population distributions of hypothetical test results for healthy and abnormal populations. *(A)* Separation is poor owing to large spread; *(B)* separation is almost perfect because spread is much smaller, even though population means are identical with *(A)*.

which misclassifies only a very small proportion of each population. Contrast this with the situation illustrated in fig 3.1B. Here the population means are exactly the same as those in fig 3.1A, because the peaks of the curves are in the same positions, but the population standard deviations are much smaller and this results in the curves being much "slimmer." Now the same decision rule is very good at separating healthy subjects from abnormal ones; only a very small proportion of subjects will be misclassified.

Thus to evaluate a proposed quantitative diagnostic test it is necessary to have information about the relative separation of the

23

population means and the sizes of the population standard deviations. Fortunately, it is not necessary to have exact information; estimates based on samples which are sufficiently large to provide a reasonable degree of precision will be adequate for all practical purposes. We hope that the reader will excuse the deliberate vagueness here, concerning what constitutes "sufficiently large" and "reasonable." This will be explained in chapter 8.

To summarise, the population mean and standard deviation are inaccessible, but they can be estimated by the *sample mean* and *sample standard deviation*, calculated from a random sample of members of the population. Statistical inference is concerned with:

(i) making statements about population means or standard deviations, based on the limited information provided by the corresponding sample values;

(ii) quantifying the uncertainty associated with these statements.

This enables statistical methods of various types to be used to assess whether for example, there is objective evidence for claiming that groups differ or that measurements are related. The practical application of this knowledge is the ability to determine whether groups of subjects differ in medically important ways or whether different types of measurements are related in ways which shed light on physiological, pathological, or biological mechanisms.

Estimating the population mean using a confidence interval

When a population is sampled, the sample mean is an estimate of the population mean. Other samples would produce different estimates and so it is important to be able to estimate the imprecision of an estimate from any given sample. Statisticians invented the term "confidence interval" to describe the range of plausible values for the population mean that are consistent with the observed sample mean.

Underlying the concept of the confidence interval is the realisation that the means of repeated samples will themselves have a distribution known as the *sampling distribution of the mean*. When the samples are selected from a normal population, the sampling distribution of the sample mean is normal with the same mean as the population, but with a standard deviation which is equal to the population standard deviation divided by the square root of the sample size. The standard deviation of the sampling distribution of the mean is called the "standard error of the mean" (SEM). Because the sampling distribution is normal, 95% of all sample means will lie within 1·96 SEM of the population mean. Given the actual value of the sample mean, the following argument produces the confidence interval for the population mean: suppose the observed sample mean is in fact one of the 95% that fall within 1·96 SEM of the population mean, then the population mean cannot be more than 1·96 SEM away from the sample mean. Consequently, the 95% confidence interval for the population mean is the range (sample mean − 1·96 SEM to sample mean + 1·96 SEM). We cannot be absolutely certain, however, that the sample mean is one of the 95% of sample means that are within 1·96 SEM of the population mean; there is a 5% chance that it is one of those that is not. So the statement "the population mean is within 1·96 SEM of the sample mean" will be correct 95 times out of 100, which is why the interval is called a 95% confidence interval. There is a minor technical difficulty as the SEM requires the population standard deviation value, which will be unknown in any practical situation. The sample standard deviation, however, can be used instead when calculating the SEM, with a correction to take into account the uncertainty arising from estimation of the population standard deviation by the sample standard deviation. This changes the number 1·96 to a somewhat larger value which depends on the sample size; it is 2·23 for samples of size 10, 2·09 for sample size 20, and 2·00 for samples of size 60 (values for all sample size may be obtained from a table of percentage points of the t-distribution.[6 12]).

Of course, there is no particular reason why the 95% probability level should be especially singled out; a higher value such as 99% might be preferable because then there is only one chance in 100 that the confidence interval fails to bracket the value of the population mean. By convention, the commonly used confidence intervals are 90%, 95%, and 99%. The higher the value selected for the probability that a given confidence level will include the population mean, the wider that interval will be. The point is illustrated as follows: 30 normal subjects were selected at random to estimate mean pO_2 in normal forearm skin, and the sample mean was 82·20 with a sample standard deviation of 8·97. Output from a Minitab analysis is shown in fig 3.2. The 95% confidence interval

25

MTB > DESCRIBE 'pO₂'

	N	MEAN	MEDIAN	TRMEAN	STDEV	SE MEAN
pO₂	30	82·20	82·38	82·05	8·97	1·64

	MIN	MAX	Q1	Q3		
pO₂	67·57	100·34	76·56	88·81		

MTB > TINTERVAL for 'pO₂'

	N	MEAN	STDEV	SE MEAN	95·0 PERCENT C.I.
pO₂	30	82·20	8·97	1·64	(78·85, 85·55)

MTB > TINTERVAL 99% for 'pO₂'

	N	MEAN	STDEV	SE MEAN	99·0 PERCENT C.I.
pO₂	30	82·20	8·97	1·64	(77·68, 86·71)

Figure 3.2   Minitab display giving basic description and 95% confidence interval for the mean tcpO₂ in forearm skin of a sample of 30 normal subjects. The first command gives the basic descriptive statistics, the second calculates by default the 95% confidence interval.

for the population mean tcpO₂ stretches from 78·85 up to 85·55; the corresponding 99% confidence interval is wider, stretching from 77·68 up to 86·71. The wider range of probable values for the population mean is the price which must be paid for being more confident that this range includes the population mean value.

Comparative investigations

Many medical research investigations entail comparisons between subjects selected from various well defined subpopulations with the aim of detecting medically or scientifically significant differences between the overall distribution of certain variables in the different subpopulations. The simplest comparative investigation involves two subpopulations which may, for example, be a population of normal controls and a population of patients with a particular disease. Such an investigation would be carried out by randomly selecting roughly the same number of subjects from each subpopulation and making the appropriate measurement on each person. We will refer to this as the *two sample comparison*. A second, similar, type of investigation is known as the *paired comparison* investigation, in which the same measurement is made on each of several subjects twice—for example, before and after treatment—and so each subject acts as his or her own control for the purpose of assessing changes brought about by treatment. You must be careful to distinguish between the two types of comparative investigation because the appropriate statistical analyses are not interchangeable.

The analysis of the two sample comparison assumes that:

(i) the measurements in each subpopulation are normally distributed;

(ii) the difference between the subpopulations manifests itself only as a difference between the corresponding population means;

(iii) the standard deviation is the same in both subpopulations.

In chapter 5 we shall describe alternative analyses to be used when these assumptions do not hold.

A confidence interval for the difference between the population means provides the answer to the question of whether the data show that the population means are different and it indicates how large the difference is likely to be.

The procedure is very similar to that used to determine a confidence interval in the single sample case. As an example, the data presented in fig 3.3 were obtained in an investigation that compared measurements of haemoglobin concentration in the blood of 80 healthy men and a similar group of 80 healthy women. The sample mean and standard deviation were 154·8 g/l and 24·9 g/l for the men, and the mean was 140·2 g/l and the standard deviation 28·1 g/l for women. The difference between the sample

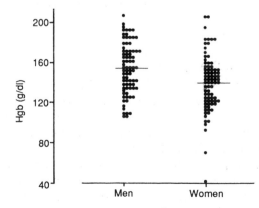

Figure 3.3   Haemoglobin concentration in men and women (80 subjects in each group).

27

means was 14·6 g/l and the standard error of this difference was 4·2 g/l. The 95% confidence interval for the difference between the population means stretches from 6·3 g/l to 22·9 g/l. This is interpreted as indicating that you can be 95% sure that average haemoglobin concentration in men can be expected to be between 6·3 g/l and 22·9 g/l higher than women. When there is only a small difference between population means—for example, in leucocyte counts, a similar investigation might produce the data illustrated in fig 3.4, with sample means of $6·97 \times 10^9/l$ and $7·04 \times 10^9/l$ and standard deviations of $1·05 \times 10^9/l$ and $0·95 \times 10^9/l$. A 95% confidence interval for the difference between the population mean for men and the population mean for women stretches from $-0·38 \times 10^9/l$ up to $0·24 \times 10^9/l$. In this case the supposition that there is no difference between the population means cannot be ruled out as zero falls inside the confidence interval.

The confidence interval is recommended as superior to *any* other method of statistical analysis in this situation because it gives a clear indication of the *size of the difference* between the population means, together with an equally clear indication of the *imprecision in our knowledge of the actual difference*. Thus there can be no doubt in the reader's mind as to whether a reported difference is medically important, because the probable size of the difference is quoted. Nor can there be much doubt about whether the sample sizes were large enough to detect worthwhile differences in an

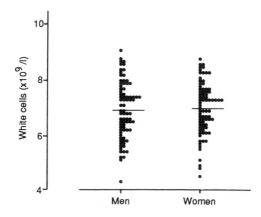

Figure 3.4   White cell counts in men and women (80 subjects in each group).

investigation which reports a "negative" finding—that is, a confidence interval which includes zero. For example, if a difference of 5 units would be medically significant but the confidence interval reported in a particular investigation stretched from −20 up to +40, its width indicates that variability is so great that a much larger investigation would be required to reduce the width of the interval to a level where you could be optimistic about detecting a difference of 5 units.

As an indication of how sample size affects the width of a confidence interval, fig 3.5 shows the end points of 95% confidence intervals for investigations with the same means and standard deviations as in fig 3.3, and calculated from samples varying in size from 10 up to 500. The gain, in terms of decreased width, from using larger sample size is quite noticeable—up to 100 per group, but declines sharply thereafter.

The analysis of results arising from a paired comparison investigation can be summarised briefly, as no new ideas are involved. Recall that two measurements are made on each subject to estimate the difference between the population means before and after treatment. The appropriate method of analysis is to subtract the first measurement from the second for each subject and calculate a confidence interval for the mean of these differences. If the

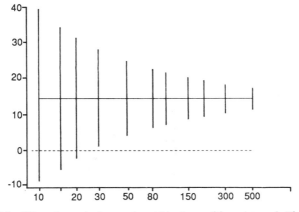

Figure 3.5 Effect of sample size on the width of a confidence interval. The bars represent confidence intervals for the difference in mean haemoglobin concentration using the means and standard deviations from the data of figure 3.3, but assuming sample sizes ranging from 10 up to 500 in each group.

confidence interval does not straddle zero, this will indicate that treatment does affect the variable of interest.

Confidence intervals compared with significance tests

There is a strong association between the confidence interval approach and an alternative commonly used in the medical literature, based on the idea of a "significance test," in which the difference between the sample means is divided by the standard error. The result is conventionally denoted by the symbol "t" and the method is known as the "*two sample t test*" (in the paired comparison, it is the mean of the differences divided by its standard error which is referred to as "t" and the corresponding test is the "*paired t test*").

The significance testing approach is based on the following argument: suppose the population means are equal, then we would expect the sample means to be roughly equal, apart from the inevitable difference resulting from sampling, and so their difference will be "close" to zero. The standard error of the difference is the appropriate scale factor for judging whether the observed difference is small enough for it to be regarded as evidence that the subpopulation means are equal. Thus "t" is the appropriate statistic for making the assessment. If "t" is large then this is taken as evidence against the supposition that the population means are equal. A "large" value is one which has a low probability of occurring when the population means are equal. This probability is called the P value in the medical literature and the significance level by statisticians.

The logic of the t test is as follows: if the P value associated with the result is small, say 0·01, then there are two possibilities:
  (i) the population means *are equal* but the investigation has produced data which have only a 1 in 100 chance of occurring or;
  (ii) the population means are not equal.
The conventional approach has been to regard an investigation as having produced evidence in favour of a genuine difference whenever the P value is less than 0·05, and then the result is reported as being "significant."

The shortcomings of the significance testing approach are well known to statisticians and have been pointed out on several occasions.[7 8] Firstly, the result of an investigation is being forced into a framework where all that matters is whether a result is or is not significant. This is surely not wise, as what really matters is whether an investigation has been able to detect a medically important difference between the population means and how large that difference is likely to be. Secondly, the significance test approach pretends that all situations can be neatly categorised as ones in which the population means are or are not exactly equal. In reality there is likely to be some difference between the population means, and so a very large investigation will stand a good chance of detecting the difference, no matter how small and medically unimportant it may be. The method can easily lead to the attitude that for example, a "significant $(P < 0.01)$" result should be interpreted as meaning that a difference which has a practical importance has been detected.

On the other hand, an investigation which results in a "not significant $(P > 0.05)$" difference risks being misinterpreted as providing conclusive evidence that a truly zero difference between the population means has been established. Nothing could be further from the truth. The correct interpretation is that any underlying difference is too small to have been detected by this particular investigation (the investigation may in fact have been too small to detect really worthwhile differences). Statistical analysis cannot be used to prove conclusively that there is absolutely no difference between a pair of population means.

By comparison the confidence interval approach is superior. As it gives a range of plausible values for the difference between the population means, the knowledgeable subject specialist is able to judge whether the difference being reported is of practical importance. In fact the confidence interval and the significance test are closely related. If the 95% confidence interval for the mean difference does not bracket zero, then the t test will produce a result which is significant at the 5% level and perhaps at an even lower level. Conversely, if the t test results in $P > 0.05$ then the 95% confidence interval will include zero, but the interval gives a more useful interpretation of the "not significant" result: the true difference may not be zero but could be any value within the interval.

As both the t test and the confidence interval approach are available in all good statistical packages it is advisable to combine the two. To illustrate this we compared the data of fig 3.3 using the "two sample" analysis from Statgraphics. The screen output is shown in fig 3.6; the major descriptive statistics for the two

31

Two sample analysis results

Sample statistics:		HbM	HbF	Pooled
	Number of obs.	80	80	160
	Average	154·817	140·238	147·528
	Variance	622·298	789·773	706·035
	Std. deviation	24·9459	28·1029	26·5713
	Median	154·9	141·9	147·7

Conf. interval for diff. in means:		95 Percent		
(Equal vars.)	Sample 1 − Sample 2	6·28021	22·8798	158 D.F.
(Unequal vars.)	Sample 1 − Sample 2	6·27931	22·8807	155·8 D.F.

Conf. interval for ratio of variances:		95 Percent	
	Sample 1 Sample 2	0·50532	1·22864

Hypothesis test for H0: Diff = 0   Computed t statistic = 3·4703
vs Alt: NE   Sig. level = 6·7024E–4
at Alpha = 0·05   so reject H0

Figure 3.6   *Screen displays produced by Statgraphics in response to a request for a two sample t test analysis of the haemoglobin data of figure 3.3.*

samples are shown in the top field. Note that both the standard deviations and the variances, which are merely the squares of the standard deviations, are displayed. Then the 95% confidence interval for the difference between the population means is given (the user can choose an alternative level such as 99%): the display next shows the results of two forms of the interval, the first being the one we have described above which assumes equal population standard deviations, the second is an alternative which is appropriate when the assumption is clearly invalid. The user may choose whichever is more appropriate, depending on the variances shown in the upper part of the panel. Thereafter the user has an opportunity for calculating a confidence interval for the ratio of the population variances at a probability level of his or her choice; this is a further guide to which of the alternative intervals to use. If the confidence interval for the ratio of the variances brackets the value one then the equal variance confidence interval is appropriate. The bottom section of the panel is written in computer statistics jargon, but we can interpret the computer output into plain English as follows: "the data provide evidence of a difference between mean haemoglobin concentrations in men and women. The difference between the sample means for two groups of 80 subjects was 14·6 g/l with a standard error of 4·2 g/l, this difference is significant

32

at $P < 0.001$, and a 95% confidence interval for the difference between healthy men and women stretches from 6·3 g/l to 22·9 g/l."

This final display can be "dumped" to the printer for a permanent record at a single key stroke. With other simple manipulations, dot plots or box and whisker plots can be displayed and recorded permanently with a graph plotter, laser printer, or ink-jet printer. A bench-based laboratory scientist can thus obtain reliable comparisons between groups of experimental observations and produce various forms of display to clarify the interpretation quickly on a microcomputer. Used properly this facility will extend the range and improve the efficiency of many types of laboratory work for a very small financial outlay.

4

Comparison of several groups: analysis of variance

Comparison of several groups where distributions approximate to normal and where variances are similar

It is unusual for a biomedical research study to involve only comparison between two groups; more often the same observation is made on each subject in several groups with the aims of (i) detecting group differences and (ii) estimating their probable magnitudes. An example of this type of study is a comparison between haemoglobin concentrations in normal men (group A), normal women not receiving medication (group B), normal women taking the contraceptive pill (group C) and women with meno-metrorrhagia (group D) (fig 4.1).

A common, but inappropriate, method of analysis of such data entails the comparison of each pair of groups using the two sample t test to make each comparison. Thus group A is compared in turn with groups B, C, and D; group B is compared with groups C and D; and finally; group C is compared with D, resulting in a total of six t tests. This approach is basically flawed because it ignores the inherent associations in multiple comparisons and will inflate the chance of obtaining a misleading result. Remember that in the t test for comparison of two groups of data, the P value is the probability of obtaining a result at least as extreme as the observed difference between the sample means when there is no difference between the corresponding population means. Consequently, when applying a single t test at a P value of 0·05, the investigator has a 5% chance of being misled into concluding that there is evidence of a difference when the population means are equal and

IMP.

34

the observed extreme result is attributable entirely to the random X variability of the responses. If two independent t tests are performed—for example, comparing A with B and C with D—in a situation where the corresponding population means are equal the probability that both will correctly indicate this is 0.95×0.95 or 0.9025 (90·25%), and so there is a 9·75% chance that at least one of the pair of tests will be misleading. If six comparisons were made (as in the haemoglobin study) and the corresponding population means were equal then the chance of a correct conclusion in all six tests is about $(0.95)^6$ or 0.735. In other words there is a greater than 1 in 4 chance that the result of at least one of the six tests will be misleading.

The probability of at least one misleading conclusion in a series of tests is known as the *error rate* of the series. The tendency for the error rate to rise rapidly as the number of groups increases means that the technique of pairwise comparisons cannot be recommended. Table 4.1 indicates the approximate error rate for comparison of several groups by pairwise t tests when it is proposed to report all results with P values of less than 0·05. Being more cautious and reporting only those results with P values less than 0·01 alleviates but does not entirely eliminate the problem.

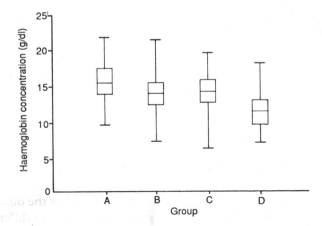

Figure 4.1 Box and whisker plots of the observed distribution of haemoglobin concentration in random samples of 100 subjects from each of the following groups: (A) healthy men; (B) healthy women not receiving medication; (C) healthy women taking the contraceptive pill; (D) women with menometrorrhagia. All distributions seem to be symmetrical and variability is about the same in all groups.

TABLE 4.1
Overall error rates when several groups are compared by performing two sample t tests on all pairs of groups

No of groups	No of pairs	Overall error rate when the chosen significance level of each test is:	
		5%	1%
3	3	14%	3%
4	6	26%	6%
5	10	40%	10%
6	15	54%	14%
10	45	90%	36%

The appropriate technique, *analysis of variance*,[34] not only takes full account of the multiple comparison nature of the problem but also uses the information in all samples to provide standard errors for the differences between pairs of population means (the pairwise *t* test method uses only information from the pair of samples being compared to determine the standard error of the difference).

The method is available in both Statgraphics and Minitab. It is based on the following assumptions: (i) the variability within each group is about the same; (ii) observed values are more or less normally distributed within each population.

The basic principle is quite simple. If there are real differences between some of the population means, this will be reflected as differences between the corresponding sample means which will be significant if the study is large enough. In any investigation involving several groups the overall variability of the responses can be separated into two components: (i) variability between sample means, indicating possible differences between population means, and (ii) variability of responses within each group, indicating natural variability within each population. If the population means are equal then differences between the sample means will be entirely due to chance variations in the individual observations within each group so that the two types of variability (i) and (ii) ought to be comparable. If there are substantial differences between the population means, however, variability between sample means (i) ought to be considerably greater than variability within groups (ii).

The analysis of variance differentiates between these situations by making a direct comparison between (i) and (ii). For technical reasons the measure of spread used is not the standard deviation but its square, the variance. The method uses (a) the variance of the set of sample means and (b) an estimate of the natural variability based on the variances of the responses in each group, known as the "pooled" within groups variance, to calculate the variance ratio, or F ratio, which is merely (a) divided by (b).

The evidence for or against differences between the population means of the various groups is assessed by determining the probability that a variance ratio at least as extreme as that actually observed could occur by chance if all the population means were equal—that is, the P value. A variance ratio which has a low P value is taken as evidence that real differences exist: by itself it does not indicate which sets are different from the remaining sets. The output from both packages is much the same and takes the form of a standard analysis of variance table (fig 4.2), which is part of the Statgraphics analysis of the data displayed in fig 4.1.

The analysis of variance is basically a significance testing procedure, so an F ratio which has a P value of less than 0·05 is conventionally taken as evidence of genuine differences between some of the population means. As usual the smaller P value the stronger is the evidence for differences. Thus in the haemoglobin example there is very strong evidence of differences between mean haemoglobin concentrations in some of the groups. Note that the analysis of variance, like all significance testing procedures, merely gives an indication of the strength of the evidence; it does not indicate which population means do differ or whether the differences are of practical, as distinct from statistical, significance.

Analysis of variance					
Source of variation	Sum of squares	d.f.	Mean square	F-ratio	Sig. level
Between groups	865·4021	3	288·4674	43·8941	0·0000
Within groups	2602·4706	396	6·5719		
Total (corrected)	3467·8727	399			

Figure 4.2   The analysis of variance table produced by Statgraphics for the data summarised in figure 4.1. F ratio is highly significant (the value 0·0000 displayed under "Sig. level" means that the P value is less than 0·00005), indicating that the data provide extremely strong evidence of differences between the population means of some groups. It is not possible to tell from this table which groups differ.

Follow up analysis

To answer such questions it is essential to report the results of a "follow up" analysis. This can be done graphically by presenting appropriate confidence intervals for the population means. There are various methods of doing this. Minitab displays individual 95% confidence intervals for the means using essentially the same method as that used for a two sample investigation, but with the important proviso that the standard error for the difference between any pair of means is derived from information on variability obtained from *all* samples and not merely from the two samples being compared. The analysis of variance and follow up produced by Minitab are displayed in fig 4.3. This shows that (i) healthy men have a higher mean haemoglobin concentration than women; (ii)

Analysis of variance   *Haemoglobin*

Source	DF	SS	MS	F
Groups	3	865·40	288·47	43·89
Error	396	2602·47	6·57	
Total	399	3467·87		

Group	N	Mean	STDEV
A	100	15·659	2·572
B	100	13·943	2·612
C	100	14·156	2·559
D	100	11·552	2·511

Pooled STDEV = 2·564

Individual 95 PCT CI's for mean based on pooled STDEV

```
- - + - - - - - - - + - - - - - - - + - - - - - - - + - - - -
                              (- - -•- -)          (- -  •  - -)
        (- - -•- -)                  (- - •  - -)
- - + - - - - - - - + - - - - - - - + - - - - - - - + - - - -
   11·2              12·6            14·0            15·4
```

Figure 4.3   The analysis of variance table provided by Minitab also includes a graphical follow up analysis. 95% confidence intervals for the population means of the four groups are interpreted in the usual way: intervals which do not overlap indicate a difference between the corresponding population means.

women taking the contraceptive pill have a mean haemoglobin concentration which cannot be distinguished from that of healthy women not receiving medication, and (iii) women with meno-metrorrhagia have a mean haemoglobin concentration that is significantly lower than that of healthy women.

The Statgraphics package produces a similar follow up analysis on request but tabulates the confidence limits rather than displaying them graphically. An extra follow up feature of Statgraphics is its ability to indicate those sample means for which there is no evidence of a difference between the corresponding population means (fig 4.4). In the section of the table headed "homogeneous groups" asterisks in the same column alongside the means for groups B and C indicate that they do not differ significantly. The technique used for these calculations is known as a *multiple comparisons procedure*[9] and several alternative methods are available within Statgraphics, differing mainly in the details of calculations involved in producing the final result. Which one is used is largely immaterial because all will give very similar results. What is important is that some form of follow up analysis should always be performed after obtaining a significant F ratio in the initial analysis of variance.

Diagnostic plots

The analysis of variance is based on assumptions of homogeneity of spread of responses in the various groups and normality of the distribution of responses. Failure of the responses to conform to these assumptions, either directly or via the presence of outliers, may result in the analysis of variance being misleading. The assumptions may be checked by examining the *residuals*, which are

Multiple range analysis for haemoglobin by group			
Method: Group	95 Percent Count	Scheffe Average	Homogeneous Groups
A	100	15·659	
C	100	14·156	*
B	100	13·943	*
D	100	11·552	

Figure 4.4   Statgraphics provides an alternative follow up analysis based on multiple comparison methods.

the deviations of the responses from the corresponding group means. The most useful plots are (i) a plot of residuals against the group means and (ii) a normal plot of the residuals (chapter 2). Residuals which are particularly large may indicate outliers. Repeating the analysis with suspect observations omitted will indicate whether they play a large part in determining the conclusions.

The plot of residuals against the group means (an additional option in Statgraphics) is very similar to the plot of the raw data which should be the starting point of the analysis of variance, except that each group of residuals is centred on zero and so visual comparison is easier. The danger sign to look out for is either one group of residuals with a much greater spread than the rest, or a tendency for the spread to vary appreciably and systemically over the groups. If either pattern appears then the assumption of uniform spread is not tenable and some corrective action such as a transformation of the data may be needed. The normal plot of the residuals should be nearly a straight line if the data conform to the normality assumption, but curvature can indicate non-normality, inhomogeneity of spread, or the presence of outliers: it is therefore wise to look at both plots. Both packages calculate residuals and fitted values on demand and so the two diagnostic plots can easily be obtained.

The broader problem of multiple testing

In many investigations various observations are made on subjects belonging to different categories and these may then be analysed in a number of ways to suggest fruitful areas for concentration of further research effort. With a large and complex data set there are likely to be several hundred ways in which various combinations of variables may be analysed. The problem of overall error rates and multiple comparisons is obviously important here, for if every result with a P value of 0.05 or less is reported as corresponding to a genuine difference, then 1 in 20 (5%) of the reported results may be misleading in the sense of indicating a difference where one does not exist. Partly, the problem arises from the use of a significance test as an exploratory tool in sifting through a large body of data: a function for which it is not ideally suited. The proportion of spuriously significant results among a large group of tests may be reduced by resisting the temptation to report *every* result with a P

value of less than 0·05, reporting instead only those results with P values of less than 0·01 or some similar figure: using 0·05 divided by the square root of the number of tests performed gives a P value which is a reasonable compromise between spurious significance and being over-stringent. Alternatively, you may adopt the viewpoint that the statistical tests performed in an exploratory situation are merely being used to generate interesting hypotheses which must be confirmed in a further investigation of at least the same size as that from which they were derived.

Replicates and repeated measures

Replicates

Whenever a method of measurement is indirect and is the result of a complex process of sample preparation it is customary for the investigator to replicate each sample. For instance, in measuring uptake of ^{3}H-TdR as an indicator of DNA synthesis it is common practice to make triplicate preparations from each sample at the same time and to measure each one. This is a recognition of the fact that the process of sample preparation and the measurement of the amount of radioactive tracer introduces quite a substantial amount of experimental variability, which is extremely difficult to control. When this is so the mean of the values from the three replicates is likely to be closer to the underlying absolute value than any one of the values. The standard deviation of the values, which may be referred to as the replicates' standard deviation, gives an indication of the variability resulting from the process of sample preparation and measurement. If the replication is performed for each subject then the replicates' standard deviation for each subject can be combined to provide a more precise measurement of experimental variability.

Information about the magnitude of the experimental variability is useful in planning further investigations but it is often incidental to the main aim of a study which is likely to be the comparison of different groups of subjects. It is therefore imperative to make a clear distinction between variability between subjects, which is used to obtain an estimate of population variability, and variability between replicates from which an estimate of experimental variability can be obtained. It is the population variability not the experimental variability which is relevant to assessing whether groups differ. When equal replication for all subjects is possible

41

then the simplest way of comparing groups is to perform an analysis of variance of the means of the replicates. When the amount of replication is not the same for each subject then a more complex analysis is required and you would be wise to consult a statistician.

Repeated measures

One form of repeated measures study involves a series of measurements made over a period of time on each one of a number of subjects in one or more groups. The type of question which the investigation is set up to answer is concerned with whether the way in which subject response changes with time differs from one group to another and, if this is so, what is it that characterises the differences. The measurements in each series, although made on the same subject, are in no sense replicates as you expect any differences between measurements made at different times to be due to changes in the absolute level of the quantity being measured and not solely attributable to experimental error as is the case with replicates.

Because a series of measurements is made on each subject, the data arising from such a study do not conform to the basic assumptions of most univariate methods of analysis which assume that each value is independent of the rest. This cannot be the case here, for a subject who starts with an initially high value is likely to continue to have high values and so the measurements on one subject will be correlated. In most cases the appropriate techniques are those of *multivariate analysis*.

Repeated measures studies are inherently more difficult to analyse and the results of the analysis are more difficult to comprehend, precisely because you are trying to understand and characterise a series of correlated measurements. It is often the case that a repeated measures study is incorrectly analysed by ignoring the fact that the measurements on a single subject are related and then using a univariate analysis of variance of the type described in this chapter. This is not recommended because it oversimplifies the true situation to such an extent that the results of the analysis are likely to be quite misleading. The correct analysis requires a familiarity with the techniques of multivariate analysis of variance and so is outside the scope of this book. The advice of your local statistical guru should be sought before embarking on a repeated measures type of study.

5

Analysis of continuous data that are not normally distributed: distribution free methods

The various statistical techniques described in the previous chapters are based on assumptions concerning the distribution of responses. In particular, outliers or extreme non-normality may seriously influence the results of any analysis which relies on the normality assumption. Normal plots of the raw data in each sample or of the residuals can be used to assess how well the data conform, provided the sample sizes are sufficiently large (chapter 2). This method is insensitive with small samples, however, as only the most extreme forms of non-normality will be detected. Fortunately, both the methods based on the t test and the analysis of variance are pretty robust as far as moderate departures from normality are concerned.

Some types of non-normality may be corrected by an appropriate transformation such as the logarithmic or the square root transformation. If a transformation to correct non-normality cannot be found, then an alternative approach is available. A significance test and the appropriate confidence interval may be determined by using distribution free (or non-parametric) methods.[10 11] These methods do not assume that the population distributions are "normal," but assume instead that the distribution shape is about the same in each population being compared.

We recommend the following procedure for deciding whether to use a distribution free procedure. First, see whether a transformation will achieve near normality. Make the transformation, and plot the transformed data looking at both the normal probability plot and the box and whisker plot. If these plots show no serious departures from normality, in other words the points on the normal plot lie more or less on a straight line and the box and whisker plot is symmetrical, then the transformation has achieved its purpose. It is therefore safe to analyse the *transformed data* by methods which are based on the assumption that the underlying distribution is normal. When reporting the results of the analysis you will have to back-transform any descriptive statistics or confidence intervals that are used so as to make them refer to the original data. If there does not seem to be a transformation which works then the data should be analysed by the appropriate distribution free method.

There is a widespread belief that distribution free methods can be applied to any data because they make no assumptions whatsoever about the underlying data distribution but this is not correct. The true state of affairs is that these methods do make some assumptions such as symmetry or that the shapes of the underlying distributions are the same. These assumptions are not so restrictive as the normality assumption, but they are implicit in the methods and must be more or less valid for the methods to be applied safely.

Distribution free equivalent of the *t* test

The median is a more appropriate indicator of location than the mean for appreciably asymmetrical non-normal distributions, so the two sample distribution free significance test assesses the evidence for a difference between the population medians: the distribution free confidence interval represents a range of plausible values for this difference.

The relevant method for *two sample comparisons* is known as the *Mann-Whitney procedure*. It is based on the principle of replacing the actual data values by their ranks. First, the two samples are combined and sorted into ascending order. Then the observations are ranked giving rank 1 to the smallest, rank 2 to the next smallest, and so on. If two or more observations are equal then the average of the ranks which would be assigned is allocated to each one.

The test statistic used to assess evidence for a difference between the population medians is the sum of the ranks in the first sample and is often designated by the letter W. The value of W reflects the relative position of the two sets of sample values. If the values in the first sample tend to be higher than those in the second sample then the larger ranks will occur predominantly in the first sample and W will be large. Obviously W will be small if the values in the first sample tend to be smaller than those in the second sample. For example, box plots of the survival times of two groups of patients with breast cancer are shown in fig 5.1. Group A comprises patients with 40% or more of malignant cells in sections of neoplastic tissue and group B patients with less than 40% of malignant cells. The plots suggest that survival may be related to percentage of malignant cells in the sense that survival seems to be somewhat longer in group B. The output from Minitab, consisting of a basic description of the data, the Mann-Whitney test, and a confidence interval for the difference between the population medians is displayed in fig 5.2. Although the median of group B is larger than that of group A, the probability of obtaining a difference in medians at least as large as this when the population medians are equal is 0·25 and consequently the difference is not significant. The conclusion is clear: the data fail to provide statistically acceptable evidence of a difference between population median survival times for the two groups.

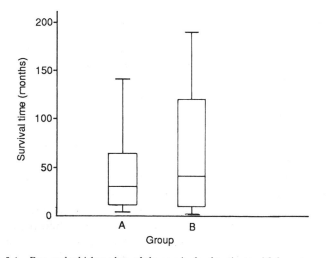

Figure 5.1   Box and whisker plots of the survivals of patients with breast cancer in a retrospective study of the use of morphometric features as predictors of survival. The distributions are extremely asymmetrical and so median survival is more informative than mean survival. This degree of asymmetry rules out the use of methods based on the normal distribution.

```
MTB > DESCRIBE 'GROUP-A' 'GROUP-B'

          N  MEAN    MEDIAN   STDEV  MIN    MAX     Q1     Q3
GROUP-A  30  39·03    30·00   35·81  3·00   142·00  10·75  64·75
GROUP-B  32  64·70    41·00   59·40  0·00   191·00   9·20 121·20

MTB > MANNWHITNEY 'GROUP-A' 'GROUP-B'

Mann-Whitney Confidence Interval and Test

GROUP-A  N = 30  MEDIAN = 30·000
GROUP-B  N = 32  MEDIAN = 41·000
POINT ESTIMATE FOR ETA1–ETA2 IS  – 11·9986
95·1 PCT C.I. FOR ETA1–ETA2 IS ( – 50, 5)
W = 862·0
TEST OF ETA1 = ETA2 VS. ETA1 N.E. ETA2 IS SIGNIFICANT AT
0·2452

CANNOT REJECT AT ALPHA = 0·05
```

Figure 5.2   Minitab display of basic descriptive statistics and the distribution free Mann-Whitney analysis of the data summarised in figure 5.1. "ETA1" and "ETA2" are Minitab jargon for the population medians for the two groups. The 95% confidence interval for the true difference between the population medians includes zero, indicating that there is insufficient evidence to claim a real difference between median survival time. This is confirmed by the P value (0·2452) associated with W. The phrase "cannot reject at alpha = 0·05" indicates that a significance test at the conventional level of 5% fails to reject the hypothesis that the population medians are equal.

The distribution free confidence interval for the difference between the population medians is based on the calculation of all the differences between the survival times for the first group and those for the second group. As this procedure is not widely known, an example of how the calculations are performed is given in the Appendix. The observed medians for the two groups are 30 months and 41 months, and you might therefore think that the best estimate of the difference between the medians of the underlying populations was merely the difference between the group medians. Unfortunately, this is not the case; the best estimate is in fact the median of all the pairwise differences between survival times. A little experimentation with some small sets of data will soon convince the reader that the difference between the medians of two groups is not the same as the median of the differences between pairs of values with one value from each group. This can be seen in fig 5.2, where the point estimate for the difference between the population medians based on the data for the two groups is − 12 months, a negative value because all the evidence seems to indicate that the population corresponding to group B has a higher median. Note, however, that the confidence interval for the difference between the population medians is -50 months up to 5 months. This can be interpreted as meaning that the data are somewhat equivocal, and can do no more than indicate that, firstly, there is a possibility that the population medians could be equal, as zero months falls within the interval, and secondly, that the population median for group B could be up to 50 months more than that of group A or could be up to 5 months less. The fact that no difference between population medians is not precluded by the confidence interval calculation is in line with the conclusion derived from the Mann-Whitney significance test. Statgraphics is not so useful in this situation; it is capable of performing the Mann-Whitney test, but does not provide the corresponding confidence interval.

A similar distribution free technique for the *paired sample comparison* is known as the *Wilcoxon technique*. Recall that a typical paired comparison investigation involves two measurements made on each subject, and the appropriate analysis involves examining the differences between the paired observations.

First, the observed differences are ordered, ignoring their signs. Ranks are then assigned in the usual way and each rank is then given the same sign as the corresponding difference. The test statistic for assessing evidence that the median of the population distribution of differences is non-zero is the sum of the signed ranks. A value close to zero indicates no real difference between the pairs of measurements, whereas a large value (positive or negative) may be evidence of genuine differences. If the P value associated with the signed rank statistic is less than 0.05 then this is taken as evidence of genuine differences between the first and second response. There is a corresponding method of calculating a confidence interval for the population median difference between the paired responses. Both Minitab and Statgraphics perform the Wilcoxon signed rank test, but only Minitab provides the confidence interval. The Appendix describes the method for calculation of the confidence interval for the benefit of Statgraphics users.

As the distribution free techniques do not take account of the actual data values, but merely their relative positions, they are much more resistant to the effects of outliers than the corresponding techniques based on the t statistic. They thus provide at least a partial remedy to the thorny problem of whether to omit apparent outliers from an analysis.

There is a common misconception that distribution free methods make no assumptions whatsoever about the data to which they may be applied and so there is a tendency to apply them in all situations, even when they are inappropriate. It is commonly stated that almost all biomedical data are non-normally distributed and so methods which have a built-in assumption of normality are of no value. This exaggerates the true situation and also ignores the fact that when data conform reasonably well with the assumption of normality, the t based techniques are not seriously misleading and are in fact slightly more *powerful*, in the sense of being able to detect smaller differences. Moreover, when they are appropriate, t based confidence intervals will be narrower than distribution free intervals. Thus our strong recommendation is to use the appropriate technique: if there is no evidence that the data are seriously out of line with the usual assumptions use the t based methods and reserve distribution free techniques for remedial cases.

Distribution free analysis of variance

As with the two sample situation, there is a distribution free technique which may be used in the event of serious non-conformity with the normality assumption, either through asymmetry or outliers which cannot be corrected. The method is the *Kruskal-Wallis test* and like the Mann-Whitney test it is based on ranks. The data from all groups are combined and ranked, then the mean rank is calculated for each group. The test statistic measures how far apart these mean ranks are and statistical theory indicates how large the Kruskal-Wallis statistic is likely to be when there are no real differences between the corresponding population medians. To illustrate the technique the Kruskal-Wallis method is applied to the haemoglobin data of fig 4.1, even though these data are normally distributed, and the corresponding output from Statgraphics is displayed in fig 5.3. The mean ranks for the four groups are somewhat different, and the extremely small P value of the Kruskal-Wallis statistic indicates that there are differences among some of the groups. Unfortunately, the utility of the Kruskal-Wallis method is somewhat reduced because neither package provides a follow up analysis and there is no easy way of obtaining distribution free confidence intervals for the group medians. One

Kruskal–Wallis analysis of haemoglobin by group		
Group	Sample size	Average rank
A	100	270·9000
B	100	204·8000
C	100	216·3000
D	100	109·9000
Test statistic = 100·5000 Significance level = 3·702E–6		

Figure 5.3   Statgraphics display for the Kruskal–Wallis analysis of the data summarised in figure 4.1. The average ranks for the four groups differ appreciably. The P value of the Kruskal–Wallis statistic T is extremely small so the analysis indicates extremely strong evidence of differences between groups which agrees with the analysis of variance and follow up analyses displayed in figures 4.2–4.4.

way round this is to apply either the signed rank method (see Appendix) to produce individual confidence intervals for each population median, or to use the Mann-Whitney based method to obtain confidence intervals for differences between all pairs of group medians.

The former is marginally simpler to apply than the latter, but either will only be useful when the sample sizes are reasonably large (more than 10 per group as a rough guide), and even in this case the procedure will tend to be rather conservative because there is nothing analogous to the residual mean square for gaining extra precision by using information from all samples in determining the standard error as in the analysis of variance. In the event of there being serious doubts about whether the standard method is applicable then the best advice is to consult your friendly, local statistical guru.

Appendix

The Mann-Whitney confidence interval for the difference between two medians

A simple example will make the method clear. Suppose two samples of responses are (in ascending order),

group A 56, 57, 58, 61, 62, 63, 66, 69 – median 61·5
group B 42, 48, 50, 51, 53, 54, 59   – median 51·0

All possible arithmetical differences between responses in group A and group B are calculated. This is most easily done by constructing a table bordered by the ordered responses with the minimum values in the "north-west" corner, entering the corresponding differences in the body of the table as shown on page 51.

The 95% confidence interval is formed by eliminating the m smallest and m largest values from this table, where the value of m is determined by consulting a table of percentage points of the Mann-Whitney distribution.[12] In this example the 10 smallest and 10 largest values must be eliminated. These values are marked with asterisks in the table. The smallest of the remaining values is 4 and the largest is 16, so the 95% confidence interval for the difference between group medians stretches from 4 to 16.

The calculations are rather tedious done by hand, but they can be shortened by noting that with the above type of tabulation the largest and smallest differences will always appear in the north-east and south-west corners of the table and so it is not necessary to calculate all differences. With a little ingenuity the calculations can be done with a spreadsheet program. Readers with some knowledge of BASIC programming should be able to construct a small program to perform the calculations.

Wilcoxon signed rank based interval

Suppose the differences between paired responses in each of 8 subjects were:

$-4, 1, 5, 7, 9, 10, 12, 16.$

The confidence interval for the median difference is obtained in a somewhat similar manner to the Mann-Whitney interval. A table is constructed, bordered by the ordered differences with the minimum value in the north-west corner, and the entries in the table are the averages of the corresponding row and column values, as shown in the calculation on page 51—for example, the entry in row 3, column 5 is $(5+9)/2 = 7$. It is necessary to complete only the upper half of the table to obtain all the necessary values because the lower half is merely a repetition of the upper portion. The 95% confidence level is obtained by eliminating the m smallest and m largest averages: the value of m is obtained from a table of the percentage points of the Wilcoxon signed ranks distribution,[12] the interval stretches from the smallest to the largest of the remaining averages. In this case the appropriate value of m is 3 and so the 95% confidence interval stretches from 1 up to 12·5.

		Group B						
		42	48	50	51	53	54	59
	56	14	8	6	5	3*	2*	−3*
	57	15	9	7	6	4*	3*	−2*
Group	58	16	10	8	7	5	4*	−1*
A	61	19*	13	11	10	8	7	2*
	62	20*	14	12	11	9	8	3*
	63	21*	15	13	12	10	9	4
	66	24*	18*	16	15	13	12	7
	69	27*	21*	19*	18*	16*	15	10

	−4	1	5	7	9	10	12	16
−4	−4·0*	−1·5*	0·5*	1·5	2·5	3·0	4·0	6·0
1		1·0	3·0	4·0	5·0	5·5	6·5	8·5
5			5·0	6·0	7·0	7·5	8·5	10·5
7				7·0	8·0	8·5	9·5	11·5
9					9·0	9·5	10·5	12·5
10						10·0	11·0	13·0*
12							12·0	14·0*
16								16·0*

6

Are variables related? Correlation and regression

Correlation

An important aspect of the statistical analysis of large quantities of measured data is the identification of patterns within the data. In this chapter elementary techniques for describing relations between pairs of continuous variables will be examined. A typical investigation will result in data which consist of measurements of several different variables on a sample of subjects. If certain variables can be shown to be related, in the sense that knowledge of the value of one variable enables an approximate value to be predicted for another, then (a) the description of the data can be simplified and (b) the fact that there is a relation may lead to interesting hypotheses about the mechanisms which cause the variables to be related.

Preliminary scatter plots should always be used to assess visually whether a pair of variables seem to be related and to indicate roughly the strength of that relation. The points on a particular plot may seem to be randomly scattered (fig 6.1A), clustered about a straight line (fig 6.1B), or a curve (fig 6.1C). Very roughly, a relation is strong if the scatter plot defines the line or curve more or less exactly with very little scatter, but is weaker if the points are more widely scattered.

The statistical measure of relation (or association) most commonly used in the biomedical literature is the *product-moment correlation coefficient*, usually abbreviated to the *correlation coefficient* and commonly denoted by the symbol "r". This is an objective measure of the strength of a linear relation between two variables and is a dimensionless number—that is, it is not affected

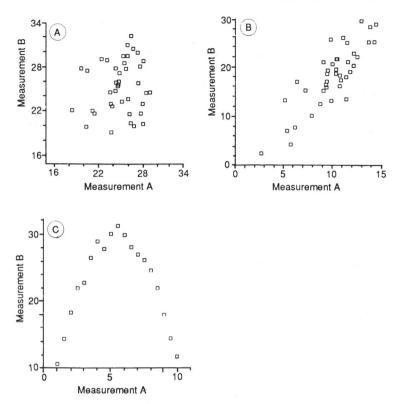

Figure 6.1   Scatter plots of hypothetical data illustrating (A) no relation between measurements A and B (r=0·129; P>0·10; (B) a linear relation between measurements A and B (r=0·84; P<0·001); (C) a curved relation between measurements A and B (r=0·021; P>0·1).

by a change of units of measurement—which always takes a value in the range –1 to + 1. The extremes of this range correspond to a perfect linear relation between the variables, a situation which will not occur in practice. It is important to realise that this type of analysis is appropriate only in situations where the relation is linear (fig 6.1B) and so it would not be correct to use it in situations similar to that illustrated by fig 6.1C where the correlation coefficient is close to zero but there is a strong non-linear relation between the measurements. With this proviso, a correlation close to zero, corresponding to a scatter plot similar to that depicted in fig 6.1A will indicate that there is no relation between the corresponding variables.

The Statgraphics correlation analysis procedure may be used to generate a table of correlations between all pairs of variables in a list entered by the user; each correlation coefficient is displayed with the corresponding sample size and P value. A similar procedure is provided in Minitab but as P values are not given a table of percentage points of the correlation coefficient must be consulted.[12] The P value relates to the test of the hypothesis of no linear relation between the variables; consequently, a correlation coefficient which was a low P value indicates the existence of a linear relation. One of the difficulties of interpreting a significant correlation is that it is difficult to form an impression of how much clustering a correlation of, say, 0·70 represents. It cannot be interpreted as about 70% of what you would expect when there is a perfect linear relation; indeed it is difficult to understand what this might mean. One solution is to look at the square of the correlation coefficient, which represents the proportion of the variability in the measured values of one variable, which is explained by its linear relation with the other variable. Thus a significant correlation coefficient of 0·7 would indicate that about 50% of the variability in one variable is explained by its linear relation with the other. Whether this is good or poor will depend on the question you are trying to answer by calculating the correlation coefficient. As we shall see later there are circumstances in which a correlation coefficient of 0·965, although highly impressive, completely fails to provide the answer to the question being posed. Whether a particular result is significant depends on the sample size: a correlation of 0·2 is significant at the 5% level if the sample size exceeds 100, yet on squaring this value we see that the supposed linear relation explains only about 4% of the variability in either variable, or to put it more forcefully, 96% of the variability is not explained. This emphasises once more that more attention should be paid to the practical (clinical or biological) meaning of a result than to statistical significance in this type of analysis.

The P value of the significance test is calculated on the assumption that the underlying population distribution of each variable is a normal distribution. The test is reasonably robust to departures from normality,[13 14] but it is not robust to the presence of outliers; a single badly placed point in conjunction with an otherwise random cloud of points can produce a highly significant correlation. This situation is illustrated in fig 6.2A; the correlation coefficient for all the data is 0·65, which is highly significant. If the outlying point is

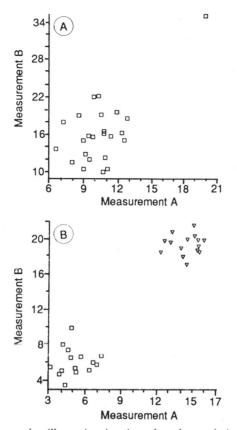

Figure 6.2 Scatter plots illustrating situations where the correlation coefficient is misleading: (A) the presence of a single outlier seriously influences the value of the correlation coefficient, with the outlier r = 0·65, omitting the outlier r = 0·07; (B) the data for men (squares) and women (triangles) fall into two separate groups. The correlation coefficient for all the data is 0·955, spuriously indicating a relation between measurements A and B. For men alone, r = 0·075 and for women alone r = 0·062, indicating that when sex is taken into account the measurements are not related.

omitted the value falls to 0·07, which is not significant. In this situation it would be most unwise to take the larger correlation as "evidence" of an association between the variables.

When data refer to two or more groups with different characteristics—for example, men and women—then the correlation coefficient may incorrectly indicate a significant linear relation between variables when the scatter plot (fig 6.2B) shows the presence of two or more separate groups within each of which the variables are not related. The spuriously significant correlation arises because the centres of the clouds of points lie on a straight line.

Rank correlation

If a scatter plot indicates a curved relation then the product-moment correlation coefficient will be inappropriate. Moderate curvature may often be removed by log-transforming one or both variables. An alternative is the *rank correlation coefficient* which may be used when the scatter plot indicates a "monotonic" curve. Monotonic means either that as the x variable increases so does the y variable, or that as the x variable increases the y variable decreases. Obviously a straight line is a special case of a monotonic "curve". The underlying curve indicated by the points in fig 6.1C is not monotonic as y first increases and then decreases as x increases. The rank correlation is the ordinary product-moment correlation calculated using the ranks of the two sets of observations when they are separately sorted into ascending order instead of the original data. The corresponding significance test does not require normality of the underlying distributions and also provides considerable protection against the malign influence of outliers. For example, the rank correlation coefficient for the data of fig 6.2A is 0·045, which is not significant; the influence of the outlying point has been attenuated.

The interpretation of a significant rank correlation is that there is a monotonic relation between the variables. There are problems of interpretation of the rank correlation coefficient similar to those encountered with the product-moment correlation coefficient; a rank correlation of 0·2 will be significant in samples of size 100 but this may not represent a practically important relation. Although not strictly valid, the interpretation of the square of the rank correlation as being an indication of the variability explained by the monotonic relation should be borne in mind.

Multiple comparisons

Correlation coefficients are generally overused and they should be avoided for anything other than exploration of the data because they are difficult to interpret correctly, and significant correlations may occur when the relation between the variables is so weak as to be practically useless.

56

Examination of a large number of variables by routine calculation of the correlations between all possible pairs, with all those which are significant at the 5% level being reported, should be avoided because this procedure is likely to be extremely misleading. For example, in a study in which 30 variables are measured on each of 200 subjects there are 435 correlations between pairs of variables ($30 \times 29/2$). Of these, you would expect 22 (5% of 435) to be spuriously significant at the 5% level and an additional 4 or 5 to be spuriously significant at the 1% level. Spuriously significant means falsely indicating an association when the corresponding pair of variables are not related. Both Minitab and Statgraphics can produce tables of correlations between all possible pairs of variables, together with the corresponding P values in the case of Statgraphics. In view of the serious problems arising from the multiple comparisons inherent in this procedure extreme care is needed in interpreting the results. The wise course is to ignore all those correlation coefficients which do not have very small P values ($0 \cdot 001$ or less); otherwise, one is likely to report and then go on to discuss and perhaps even provide speculative explanations for a large number of spuriously significant correlations.

Linear regression analysis

Linear regression analysis is a powerful and widely applicable technique for fitting straight lines or certain types of curves to data and assessing how well the fitted model describes the data. The method is used to fit a linear relation between two variables, one of which is known as the *response variable*, or y variable, the other being referred to as the *explanatory variable*, or x variable.

The decision as to which variable is the response and which is explanatory depends on the context of the investigation. Sometimes it is quite obvious which is which. For example, in looking at changes over time (fig 6.3), where acinar volume is plotted against age, it is clear that age must be the explanatory variable. In an investigation of the response of PHA stimulated lymphocytes to different concentrations of a particular steroidal drug, concentration must be the explanatory variable. In other situations the decision may not be so clear cut, the relation between height and weight in a group of subjects of the same age and sex being a classic example. Depending on the purpose of the investigation there could be two objectives; given a subject's height you might want to

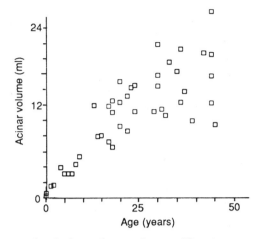

Figure 6.3   Scatter plot of acinar volume against age. There is some suggestion of curvature and an obvious indication that variability increases with age.

say something about their likely weight, or given a subject's weight you might want to predict their likely height. In the first situation it is sensible to take height as the explanatory variable, but in the second, height should be taken as the response variable.

In using simple linear regression analysis the aim is to explain at least part of the variability in the response variable values by means of the model:

$$\begin{bmatrix} \text{value of} \\ \text{response} \\ \text{variable} \end{bmatrix} = \text{intercept} + \text{slope} \times \begin{bmatrix} \text{value of} \\ \text{explanatory} \\ \text{variable} \end{bmatrix} + \begin{bmatrix} \text{unexplained} \\ \text{residual} \\ \text{amount} \end{bmatrix}$$

The various parts of this model are illustrated in fig 6.4. The intercept and slope are often referred to as the parameters of the line. It must be emphasised that this is only the simplest of the regression models available for relating values of a response variable to values of explanatory variables; polynomial regression may be used to fit curved relations and multiple regression may be used to find a small set of explanatory variables which together provide a good prediction of a response.

The model assumes that the values of the explanatory variable are known exactly; examples of variables for which this condition is likely to be true are age, volume of an organ or tumour

58

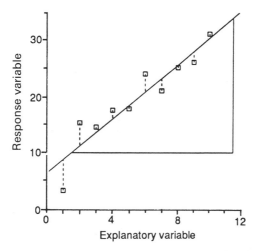

Figure 6.4   Diagram illustrating the components of the linear regression model. The slope of the fitted line is the ratio of two sides of the triangle (vertical/horizontal), the intercept is the value of the response predicted by the fitted line when the value of the explanatory variable is zero, the broken lines joining the data points to the fitted line indicate the residuals.

determined after excision, body weight and basically all measurements of quantities which show long term stability made directly with some instrument that has extremely small instrumental error. The component labelled "unexplained residual amount" in the model may be due to instrumental error in the measurement of the response variable, or it may represent biological variability between subjects who happen to have the same value for the explanatory variable, or it may be a combination of both.

As an example, we shall consider an investigation of the relation between total volume of the acinar units in the normal thyroid gland and age. Ideally, such a study should be conducted by measuring the response variable for equal numbers of subjects at each chosen age point as both the average level and the variability of the response variable may be related to age. The data displayed in fig 6.3 are therefore less than ideal because early ages are underrepresented but they will serve to illustrate the essentials of the analysis. Visual inspection shows that there is a clear relation between acinar volume and age, but variability also seems to be related to age. The output of the Statgraphics simple linear

Regression analysis – Linear model: $Y = a + bX$				
Dependent variable: avol			Independent variable: age	
Parameter	Estimate	Standard error	T value	Prob. level
Intercept	2·89593	0·993577	2·94428	5·2562E–3
slope	0·341179	0·0369029	9·24533	1·10669E–11
Analysis of variance				
Source	Sum of squares	Df	Mean square	F ratio	Prob. level
Model	937·25108	1	937·25108	85·47606	·00000
error	460·53296	42	10·96507		

Total
(corr.)   1397·7840   43
Correlation coefficient = 0·818857   R-squared = 67·05 percent
Stnd. error of est. = 3·31135

Figure 6.5   Statgraphics display of the results of fitting a straight line to the data of figure 6.3.

regression module for these data is shown in fig 6.5. Interpretation of the top part of the table is straightforward. The fitted linear relation is:

$$\text{acinar volume} = 2·90 + 0·34 \times \text{age}$$

while the standard errors indicate the precision of the corresponding parameters and provide the information needed for tests of the hypotheses that the population intercept and slope are zero. Under the heading "T value" are the estimates divided by their standard errors, the values under "Prob. level" indicate the probability of obtaining t values as extreme as those observed in a situation where the corresponding population parameter is zero. As in most situations where the scatter plot indicates an association the investigator will expect the slope to be non-zero, this t test is not very informative unless zero turns out to be a plausible value for the slope, in which case the conclusion would be that the data contain no evidence of a linear relation between the variables. Confidence intervals are usually more informative and take the form

$$\left[\begin{array}{c} \text{parameter} \\ \text{estimate} \end{array} \right] \pm \left[\begin{array}{c} \text{standard} \\ \text{error} \end{array} \right] \times \left[\begin{array}{c} \text{percentage point of} \\ \text{the } t \text{ distribution} \end{array} \right]$$

The 95% confidence interval for the slope is obtained by looking up the 5% point of the t distribution in a set of statistical tables; the number of degrees of freedom required is shown in the Statgraphics output in the row labelled "Error" under the "Df" column (42 in this case). In this example the percentage point value is 2·02 and so the 95% confidence interval for the slope parameter stretches from 0·27 to 0·42.

The analysis of variance table divides the total variability in the response values, which is the value under "Sum of Squares" in the row labelled "Total" into components attributable to the model and the unexplained residual. The "mean squares" are the corresponding sums of squares divided by their degrees of freedom and the "F ratio" is the model mean square divided by the error mean square. In this example the F ratio is large and the value under "Prob. level" indicates that the chance of getting so large an F ratio is very small if there is no relation between acinar volume and age. Accordingly, we may conclude that the data provide extremely strong evidence of a relation. The correlation coefficient needs no explanation, more informative is the value labelled "R-squared" which is the square of the correlation coefficient and indicates that 67% of the variability in acinar volume can be explained by the linear relation with age.

A further useful graphical display generated on request by Statgraphics is shown in fig 6.6. As the fitted line is estimated from a sample of 44 subjects there will be some uncertainty about the true average acinar volume at any age. The curves close to the fitted line indicate the 95% confidence band for the average acinar volume. As well as this you may well be interested in predicting what the actual acinar volume (as distinct from the average value) would be for a new subject of a specified age. The outer lines (which are symmetrical about the fitted line) indicate the 95% prediction limits and bracket the predicted value in 95 cases out of 100. Note that these are quite wide, a consequence of the considerable biological variability in the data; note also that at age 12 or less the lower prediction limit will be negative, which is clearly impossible. This indicates that a straight line with constant residual variability may not be the most sensible way of fitting these data.

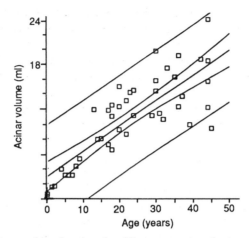

Figure 6.6   Statgraphics plot of results of linear regression of acinar volume on age. The inner curves indicate the 95% confidence band for the average acinar volume. The outer lines are the 95% prediction limits for actual acinar volume.

Underlying assumptions in regression analysis

In common with other statistical methods, simple linear regression analysis makes several assumptions which should be checked before accepting the results of the analysis. The assumptions are:

(i) the relation is linear;

(ii) the spread of the data about the line is the same at all levels of the explanatory variable;

(iii) the deviations of the data values from the line are normally distributed.

These assumptions can be checked visually with statistical packages by making diagnostic plots of the residuals which are the differences between the observed values of the response variable and the corresponding fitted values. To detect departures from linearity a plot of the residuals against the fitted values is useful. The danger sign is an obvious pattern such as a trend or pronounced curvature.

The same type of plot can be used to detect failure of assumption (ii)—if the points appear to fan out in a wedge then this indicates uneven spread. In either case more advanced techniques of regression analysis may be used to overcome the problem.

A normal plot of the residuals (chapter 2) can be used to check the assumption of normality, although it suffers from the problem that failure of either of the other assumptions can cause the plot to be curved rather than straight. Outliers can also cause problems as they will tend to pull the fitted line towards themselves, particularly if they appear near the extremes of the range of the explanatory variable. Any observation with a particularly large residual should be examined to ensure that it is not erroneous or in some way atypical. Comparing fits with and without suspected outliers will give an indication of their importance in determining the parameters of the line.

In the Minitab package observations which have large residuals or have a large influence on the fitted line are automatically indicated. Statgraphics has similar facilities, including the ability to remove points one at a time and assess the effect of this on the fitted line. If the diagnostic plots indicate that the data do not conform to one or more of the standard assumptions then there are methods for alleviating the problem. If the relation is non-linear then a transformation may provide the remedy. Log transforming either or both the response and explanatory variable(s) may be tried.

The residual plot in fig 6.7 shows curvature and fanning, indicating that the relation is perhaps curved and that variability

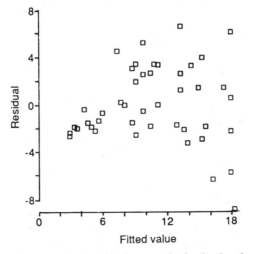

Figure 6.7   Diagnostic plot of the residuals versus the fitted values for the regression of acinar volume on age. There is a strong pattern (curvature and fanning) which indicates that a linear relation with constant residual variability is not an adequate description of the data.

increases with age. Logarithmic transformation of both variables before fitting a straight line to the log-transformed data is useful here. In this example this leads to the estimated relation:

$$\log(\text{acinar volume}) = 0{\cdot}356 + 0{\cdot}49 \times \log(\text{age}),$$

accounting for 86·9% of the variability in the log-transformed volumes. This can then be back-transformed to give the relation:

$$\text{acinar volume} = 2{\cdot}27 \times \text{age}^{0{\cdot}49},$$

for which the Statgraphics plot is shown in fig 6.8. Note that the relation is curved (volume is almost proportional to the square root of age), and that the 95% prediction limits are also curved and diverge with increasing age, which accords more with the pattern of the data.

It must be emphasised that the results of regression analysis can be used validly to predict the size of a response variable for a given value of explanatory variable only within the limits of the range of explanatory variable values used in deriving the regression equation. Any extrapolation is extremely hazardous because it relies on the assumption that the fitted relation holds outside the given range. Acinar volume, for instance, tends to decrease for ages

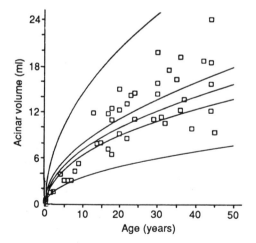

Figure 6.8 *Statgraphics plot of the relation obtained by log-transforming both acinar volume and age before regression analysis. The fitted relation is curved as are the 95% confidence limits (inner curve) and 95% prediction limits (outer curves).*

above about 55 years and so neither of the fitted regression equations could be used to predict acinar volumes for ages above 45 years.

Misuse of correlation and regression in method comparison studies

When a new method of measurement is developed it is usual to compare it with the standard method to decide whether it can replace the older method. This is done by making the same measurement by both methods on each of a number of subjects. The important question is whether the measurements agree. Basically the situation is as follows: for each subject there is an unknown true value, so when a measurement is made by a particular method the result will differ from the true value by a measurement error for that particular method. Measurement error varies from one subject to another and is likely to differ between methods. The *precision* of a method is determined by making a number of measurements on the same subject—that is, of the same true value—provided that the true value is stable over the period required to make all the measurements. The standard deviation of the results is a measure of the precision of the method. A method is accurate if the measurements cluster around the true value, and consequently the *accuracy* of a method can only be determined in situations where the true value is known. A series of repeated measurements of the unknown true value for a given subject cannot determine the accuracy of a method.

In comparing two methods of measurement it is important to determine whether they are (a) equally accurate and (b) equally precise. The starting point of the analysis should be a scatter plot of the data as shown in fig 6.9, which refers to a comparison of measurements of thyroid stimulating hormone concentration (TSH) by radioimmunoassay (RIA) and fluorescence immuno-assay (FIA). Note that the "identity line," which has unit slope and zero intercept, is included to provide a guide to interpretation of the plot. Most of the points fall below this line, indicating that the two methods do not agree; note also that there seem to be problems with measurements of low concentations.

The correlation coefficient is often misused as a way of analysing such data, typically the correlation coefficient will be very high (0·965 in this example) and this is misinterpreted as confirming

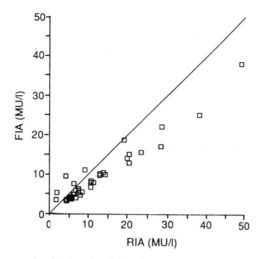

Figure 6.9 Scatter plot showing the relation between values obtained by two methods of measurement of thyroid stimulating hormone. Most points fall below the identity line, suggesting a constant proportionate difference between the methods. Some points at low concentration seem rather erratic.

that the methods agree. This is wrong as the correlation coefficient measures the strength of the relation between the results by the two methods, not whether they tend to agree. A set of measurements which cluster closely around any line, as would occur if one method were to produce results which were on average only 25% of the values given by the other, will result in a high correlation coefficient. As the methods have been developed to measure the same quantity they would be expected to produce measurements which are related.

Closer examination of the problem suggests that methods are likely to disagree in one of two ways: (a) the values will differ on average by a constant amount; (b) the values produced by one method will be on average a fixed percentage of those given by the other—that is, a constant proportionate difference. In case (a) the points will tend to cluster around a line which is parallel to the identity line, whereas in case (b) the points will cluster around a line which has a non-unit slope.

These observations form the basis of a regression method of analysis. If the confidence interval for the slope of the regression line includes the value one then case (b) is eliminated and so the confidence interval for the intercept is examined and if it brackets zero then case (a) is also eliminated and the conclusion is that the methods agree. There is, however, an objection to this method because as both sets of measurements are of unknown true values subject to varying amounts of error there are two regression lines which can be fitted, depending on which method is chosen as the explanatory or x variable. For example, taking RIA as the explanatory variable gives the line;

$$FIA = 0\cdot95 + 0\cdot69 \times RIA$$

with confidence intervals $(0\cdot63, 0\cdot75)$ for the slope and $(-0\cdot01, 1\cdot90)$ for the intercept. Taking FIA as the explanatory variable results in:

$$RIA = -0\cdot47 + 1\cdot36 \times FIA$$

with confidence interval $(1\cdot24, 1\cdot48)$ for slope and $(-1\cdot87, 0\cdot93)$ for intercept. In this case the conclusion is relatively straightforward as neither line is parallel to the identity line, the methods differ by a constant proportionate amount. If one or both methods are imprecise, however, the confidence intervals may be very wide, leading to the possibly erroneous conclusion that the methods agree. In fact, the greater the imprecision the more likely you are to decide that the methods are in agreement using the regression method. With somewhat greater precision the regression method may be equivocal. Take, for example, the case of the hypothetical data illustrated in fig 6.10. If method A is chosen as the explanatory variable the 95% confidence interval for the slope is $(0\cdot72, 0\cdot95)$, which seems to indicate a constant proportionate difference, but with method B as the explanatory variable the slope confidence interval is $(0\cdot94, 1\cdot24)$ and the intercept interval is $(-30\cdot0, 19\cdot9)$, suggesting that the methods agree.

An extremely simple method of analysis has been proposed by Altman and Bland,[15][16] and this is more informative than the regression method. As the differences between corresponding measurements contain the information needed to decide whether the methods agree, the most sensible approach is to analyse these differences. To decide between the cases of constant difference and constant proportionate difference, the difference between each pair of measurements is plotted against the average of the pair. If the methods agree then the average of a pair is the best estimate of the

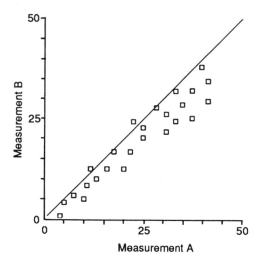

Figure 6.10   Scatter plot of hypothetical data which produces contradictory results if regression analysis is used in an attempt to assess the degree of agreement between the two methods of measurement.

corresponding true value and there ought to be no relation between the differences and averages; the scatter plot should show a random cloud of points and the correlation coefficient should not be significant. This will also be true if the methods differ by a constant amount. If the methods differ by a constant proportionate amount, however, then differences between measurements corresponding to smaller true values. The plot will then show a significant linear relation with a significant correlation coefficient. This is the case for the TSH comparison (fig 6.11A).

When methods differ by a constant amount the 95% confidence interval for the mean of the differences indicates the likely size of the difference between the methods. If methods differ by a constant proportionate amount then you should log-transform the raw data and work with the average and difference of the pairs of log-transformed values. When the TSH data are treated in this way most of the points lie in a horizontal band with a few outlying points corresponding to the samples where there were difficulties of measurement at low concentration (fig 6.11B). The rank correlation, used to attenuate the influence of the outliers, between the differences and averages is 0·17 which is not significant $(P > 0·1)$. The median difference (outliers again) is 0·13 and the distribution free confidence interval (chapter 5) for the median difference

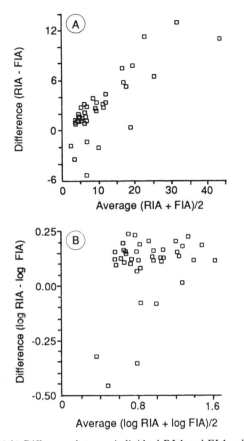

Figure 6.11   (A) Differences between individual RIA and FIA values plotted against their averages. There is clearly a linear relation between differences and averages (rank correlation = 0·704, P < 0·01), indicating that there is a constant proportionate difference between the two methods of measurement. (B) Differences between logarithms of individual RIA and FIA values plotted against averages of their logarithms. Most points lie in a horizontal band (rank correlation 0·171, P > 0·1) confirming that there is a constant proportionate difference between the two methods of measurement.

stretches from 0·10 up to 0·15. Back-transforming this interval we can say that FIA values are likely to be between 71% and 79% of those given by RIA, except at low concentrations where at least one of the methods is very unreliable.

7

Analysis of categorical data

Analysis of counts and proportions

The previous chapters in this book have been concerned with the analysis of data measured on an objective scale ("continuous" data). There are, however, many occasions when some or all of the data are collected as *nominal variables*—that is, something which may fall into one of a set of named categories and is not ordinarily measured—or as *ordinal data*—that is, a feature which can be ranked subjectively by the observer but not measured objectively, as, for example, the severity of an illness. Thus nominal variables arise when each patient may be assigned to one of several mutually exclusive categories distinguished by names—for example, the sex of a patient is either male or female, and there is no meaningful way of ordering such categories. In contrast, an ordinal variable involves a set of mutually exclusive categories which can be sensibly ordered, such as the staging or grading of a neoplasm into categories of increasing extent of disease or greater apparent aggressiveness.

Nominal data may be coded—for example, male = 1, female = 2—but the coding is an arbitrary label because the numerical values chosen as codes have no intrinsic meaning. Ordinal data are commonly coded with the simplest series of ascending integers—for example, none = 0, mild = 1, moderate = 2, severe = 3—as the integers 0,1,2,3 preserve the relative ordering of the categories—but any other ascending series could be used, as such as none = 0, mild = 6, moderate = 20 and severe = 500. It is essential to remember that the actual increments in the ordinal series (none, mild, moderate, severe) are probably unequal and so when using a coding such as 0,1,2,3 it would be quite improper to assume that "2" was twice as far up the grading scale as "1." It is for this reason that descriptive statistics such as the sample mean and standard deviation should not be used to summarise either nominal or ordinal data (the average sex of a sample of subjects is meaningless).

There are two special situations where data are commonly encountered as counts or proportions. The first concerns measurements using radioactive tracers such as uptake of ^{3}H-TdR as an indicator of DNA synthesis. Here the counts are expressed as counts per minute (cpm) and are often large. The second arises when particular features are counted directly as in enumeration of blood cells or point counting in histometric methods. In both cases relatively large numbers are counted and there will be as many counts or proportions as there are specimens. Consequently, it is often possible to treat the data is if they were true measurements on a continuous scale, but care must be taken to ensure that the data conform to the basic assumptions of the chosen statistical methods of analysis which were devised for measured data.

Estimating a single proportion

It is very unlikely that the sole purpose of an investigation would be the estimation of a single proportion—for example, the proportion of leprosy cases showing the lepromatous form of the disease in a particular country—but it is instructive to look at this example to appreciate some of the limitations of estimation when dealing with proportions. The investigation would proceed by taking a random sample of cases and classifying each one as either lepromatous or not. Thus in 250 cases there might be 175 lepromatous and 75 non-lepromatous so that the estimate (p) of the population proportion would be 175/250 or 0·7. To calculate the 95% confidence interval, as a measure of the precision of this estimate, it is necessary to obtain the standard error of the estimate by substitution of the value of the estimate in the formula:

$$\text{SE of a proportion} = \sqrt{(p(1-p)/n)}$$

and so in this case the standard error is $\sqrt{(0·7 \times 0·3/250)} = 0·029$. The critical value used in calculating the 95% confidence interval is 1·96. By using the formula:

$$\text{estimate} \pm \text{critical value} \times \text{SE of estimate,}$$

71

it is clear that the 95% confidence interval for the proportion of patients with leprosy showing the lepromatous form of the disease stretches from 0·643 up to 0·757, with the usual interpretation that there is a 95% chance that the population percentage could be as low as 64·3% or as high as 75·7%.

This method of calculation of the 95% confidence limits is valid only when the sample size is reasonably large. For very small sample sizes, say 30 or less, the confidence interval can be read directly from a chart given in Neave's tables[12]—for example, if the estimated value of the proportion is 0·7 based on a sample of 10 then Neave's tables give 95% confidence limits stretching from 0·35 up to 0·88. Under these conditions misuse of the formula would give the interval as 0·42 up to 0·98. Notably, the correct interval is not symmetrical about the estimated value of 0·7, but both intervals are so wide as to be virtually useless. This example emphasises how little reliance can be placed on estimates of proportions based on small samples of cases.

One very simple way of assessing the sample size needed to achieve a given precision is to specify the width of confidence interval which is acceptable before the start of the investigation. For example, if the investigator has prior knowledge from reports of similar investigations that the proportion is likely to be around 0·4 and a 95% confidence interval of width 0·1 is required, as the width is twice the critical value multiplied by the standard error of the estimate then:

$$\text{width} = 2 \times 1\cdot96 \times \sqrt{(p(1-p)/n)}.$$

Introducing the prior estimate $p = 0\cdot4$ into this formula results in the equation:

$$0\cdot1 = 3\cdot92 \times \sqrt{(0\cdot24/n)}$$

for which the solution is $n = 369$. This is quite a lot larger than might be anticipated by an inexperienced investigator and shows how much effort is needed to get even moderately precise estimates of proportions.

This calculation requires prior knowledge of the probable size of the proportion which the investigation is supposed to estimate; if it is not possible to make a reasonable guess at this value then $p = 0\cdot5$ should be substituted in the formula relating width to sample size as the standard error takes it maximum value when $p = 0.5$. This gives the simple result:

$$n = (1.96/\text{width})^2$$

for calculating the sample size required for a 95% confidence interval of a given width. This approach will err on the side of caution but will avoid unwarranted optimism in planning investigations.

Comparison of two proportions

It is valid to compare the proportions showing a given character only when the samples have been selected randomly from two populations. In general the sample sizes need not be equal, but it is best if they are not too dissimilar. Bearing in mind the imprecision inherent in estimates of proportions from small samples it would not be sensible to sample 200 subjects from one population and only 20 from the other if a precise estimate of the difference between the proportions was required.

Table 7.1 gives the results of a comparison of the prevalence of the Km 1 immunoglobulin allotype in patients with pulmonary tuberculosis and healthy controls in Indonesia. The Km 1 allotype is present in 32% of the patients and in 57% of the controls. It is more important to determine a confidence interval for the difference between the population proportions than to perform a significance test to determine whether the data provide evidence of a significant difference between the population proportions. The first of these procedures is obviously more informative because it is concerned with practical significance; the second may lead us into the trap of mistakenly emphasising statistical significance.

TABLE 7.1
Comparison between prevalence of Km 1 immunoglobin allotype in Indonesian patients with pulmonary tuberculosis and healthy controls

	Km 1 positive	Km 1 negative	Total
Patients	39	82	121
Controls	72	60	132
Total	111	142	253

The χ^2 *test* is a significance testing procedure which is appropriate in various situations where categorical data must be analysed.[3] In this particular example it provides a test of the hypothesis that the proportion of subjects with the Km 1 allotype is the same in patients and controls. The test is based on a comparison of what would be expected if this were the case with what is actually observed. As a working hypothesis, suppose that the proportion of subjects with the Km 1 allotype is the same in both populations, then the information in the two samples may be combined to give 111/253, or 0·4387 as the best estimate of this proportion. On average, 43·87% of subjects in each sample would be expected to bear the Km 1 allotype—that is, 53·08 patients and 57·91 controls —and by similar reasoning 67·92 patients and 74·09 controls would not be expected to carry the Km 1 allotype. These are the *expected counts* and they should be interpreted as long run averages; it is clearly impossible to observe fractions of one subject. The overall discrepancy between the observed and expected counts is known as the χ^2 *statistic* and is the sum over the four "cells" of the table of the values of:

$$(\text{observed count} - \text{expected count})^2 / \text{expected count}.$$

Regrettably, both Minitab and Statgraphics concentrate on significance testing and ignore estimation. The Minitab output for the χ^2 test is displayed in fig 7.1. The χ^2 value of 12·765, which has a *P* value of 0·0004, indicates that there is extremely strong evidence that the proportion of subjects bearing the Km 1 allotype is not the same in the population of patients with pulmonary tuberculosis as it is in the population of healthy controls.

It is a simple matter to produce a table similar to table 7.1 using Statgraphics. Suppose that the relevant data are stored as two variables, "type" and "Km 1", in a file. The "type" variable contains, for each subject, either the value 1 indicating a patient, or the value 2 indicating a control subject. In the same way the "Km 1" variable contains, for each subject, either the value 1 indicating a Km 1 positive test result, or the value 2 indicating a Km 1 negative test result. The cross-tabulation option produces a table which shows how many patients and how many controls are Km 1 positive and how many are Km 1 negative. The input screen setting up the cross-tabulation is shown in fig 7.2 and this produces the table shown in fig 7.3. Note that the values below the counts are percentages and not expected counts. A further screen displays the results of the χ^2 test (fig 7.4). The phrase "with Yates' correction" refers to a particular correction which was originally suggested by the statistician Frank Yates as an attempt to improve the applicability of the χ^2 distribution to the analysis of discrete data. Its use is

```
MTB > NAME C1 'KM1 +'
MTB > NAME C2 'KM1 -'
MTB > CHISQ 'KM1 +' 'KM1 -'

Expected counts are printed below observed counts

              KM1 +    KM1 -    Total
      1         39       82      121
              53·09    67·91

      2         72       60      132
              57·91    74·09

Total          111      142      253

ChiSq =  3·738 + 2·922 +
             3·427 + 2·679 = 12·765

df = 1

MTB > CDF 12·765;
SUBC> CHISQ 1.
     12·7650     0·9996

MTB > NOTE: So the p value is 1 - 0·9996 = 0·0004
```

Figure 7.1   Minitab output for the χ^2 analysis of incidence of the Km 1 immunoglobulin allotype (table 7.1). CDF command is used to determined the P value of the χ^2 statistic.

```
        Data vector A:                    Km1
          Labels A:           2 4 RESHAPE 'Km1 + Km1 -'
        Data vector B:                    type
          Labels B:         2 8 RESHAPE 'patientscontrols'
        Percentages:                     Rowwise
```

Figure 7.2   Input screen to obtain Statgraphics cross-tabulation of variables "Km 1" and "type". The label fields contain the specification of the labels for individual rows and columns of the table. 2 4 RESHAPE 'Km 1 + Km 1 -' indicates that the quoted text is to be split into two labels each consisting of four characters. The "rowwise" option has been chosen for percentages, indicating that the values in each row are to be expressed as a percentage of the row total as well as being displayed as row counts.

Cross-tabulation of Kml by type			
Kml type	Kml+	Kml−	Row total
Patients	39 32·2	82 67·8	121 47·8
Controls	72 54·5	60 45·5	132 52·2
Column total	111 43·9	142 56·1	253 100·0

Figure 7.3   Cross tabulation of the variables "Km 1" and "type" produced by Statgraphics. Note that the lower values in each cell are percentages not expected counts.

Summary statistics for contingency tables			
Chi-square	D.F.	Significance	
12·7651	1	3·53145E–4	
11·8750	1	5·68912E–4	with Yates correction
Statistic	Symmetric	With rows dependent	With columns dependent
Lambda	0·14655	0·18182	0·10811
Uncertainty coeff.	0·03702	0·03684	0·03720
Somer's D	−0·22462	−0·22611	−0·22314
Eta	0·22462	0·22462	0·22462

Figure 7.4   Statgraphics output for the χ^2 analysis of the Km 1 immunoglobulin allotype (table 7.1). The P value for the test is 0·0004 to four decimal places.

somewhat controversial as several studies have indicated that it does not always bring about the desired improvement. It is probably best ignored and certainly should not be used as an argument for nudging a marginally significant result in a direction favoured by the investigator.

Statgraphics is less satisfactory than Minitab as it does not give the expected counts. Statgraphics also gives, in the lower half of the display, several statistics which are irrelevant to the problem of testing whether two population proportions are equal. The various statistics labelled "Lambda", "Uncertainty Coeff", "Somer's D", and "Eta" are all equivalents of the correlation coefficient for counted data and indicate the extent to which the variables used to construct the cross-tabulation are related or associated. This is irrelevant in this particular situation where the question of interest is whether the population proportions differ, and not whether Km 1 allotype is related to a subject's status as a patient or a control. To be fair to Statgraphics, the χ^2 test is an "all-purpose test" which can be used to investigate a rather confusing number of different situations, as we shall see, and as the authors of the package can never be sure of the circumstances under which any particular user is applying the test, they have played safe and produced a selection of potentially useful statistics. This illustrates something which the intelligent user of a statistics package should always bear in mind: the fact that certain statistics are automatically produced by the computer does not mean they are necessarily relevant.

The next and more important step is to calculate a confidence interval so as to interpret the result of the χ^2 test. Unfortunately, neither package does this, but it is quite easy to calculate the 95% confidence interval using the formulae given in the Appendix. The result of the investigation may be summarised as follows: the proportion of patients with pulmonary tuberuclosis bearing the Km 1 allotype is estimated to be 32·3% with a standard error of 4·2%, and for normal controls the proportion is 54·5% with a standard error of 4·3%; this difference is highly significant ($\chi^2 = 12·765$; $P = 0·0004$), and the 95% confidence interval for the difference indicates that the proportion of patients bearing the Km 1 allotype is likely to be between 10·4 and 34·2 percentage points lower than the corresponding proportion for healthy controls.

If the sample sizes are very small then a problem may arise. Suppose that we try to analyse the hypothetical data in table 7.2 which correspond to a drastically scaled down version of the previous investigation. Minitab produces the display shown in fig 7.5: note the warning message "2 cells with expected counts less than 5·0", which indicates that the sample sizes are too small for the χ^2 test to be reliable. The general rule is that the test is reliable only when all *expected* counts are greater than 5. Note that the rule refers to expected counts, it is quite in order to apply the test when some observed counts are less than 5, provided that all expected counts exceed 5. There is a test known as *Fisher's exact test* which can be used in this situation and details of which are given in the Appendix. Statgraphics automatically performs the exact test whenever the χ^2 test is likely to be invalid.

The best advice that can be given here is that the investigator should avoid getting into this situation by keeping sample sizes reasonably large. When an investigation aims to compare proportions which are expected to be very small expert advice should be sought, as it is likely that extremely large sample sizes will be needed to obtain worthwhile data and this may involve multicentre collaboration or data collection over a long period of time. In such circumstances diagnostic criteria, laboratory procedures, and record keeping systems must be carefully standardised, and active quality control of the results, perhaps by means of periodic quality audits will be essential.

Comparison of several proportions

Comparison of several samples from different populations to detect and estimate differences between proportions is dealt with by a straightforward extension of the χ^2 method. The situation is analogous to that in which the analysis of variance is used for measured data, so a single significance test is first applied to all of the data to assess the evidence for any differences between the population proportions, and a follow up investigation determines which proportions are different: the problem of multiple comparison analogous to that seen with measured data (chapter 4) arises in the follow up stage.

Table 7.3 shows the results of Leprosin A skin testing in healthy controls, two groups of patients with leprosy, and two groups of contacts of leprosy victims. The relevant questions here are

TABLE 7.2
Hypothetical results of much smaller investigation of prevalence of Km 1 allotype

	Km 1 positive	Km 1 negative	Total
Patients	2	5	7
Controls	7	6	13
Total	9	11	20

```
MTB > CHISQUARE C1 C2

Expected counts are printed below observed counts
              C1        C2      Total
    1          2         5        7
             3·15      3·85
    2          7         6        13
             5·85      7·15
  Total        9        11        20
ChiSq = 0·420 + 0·344 +
        0·226 + 0·185 = 1·174
df = 1
2 cells with expected counts less than 5·0
```

Figure 7.5 Minitab output for the χ^2 analysis of the data shown in table 7.2. The warning about expected count less than 5 indicates that the χ^2 test may be misleading.

concerned with whether there are differences between the responsiveness of subjects in the various groups to Leprosin A. The Minitab output is shown in fig 7.6, with expected counts calculated on the same principle as before; there are a total of 149 positive responses in 253 subjects, so if there were no differences between the rates of positive response in the various subpopulations the best estimate of the common rate of positive responses is 149/253, or 0·589, so 58·9% of each sample might be expected to show a positive skin test and 41·1% to show a negative response. The χ^2 statistic is calculated by summing:

$$(\text{observed count} - \text{expected count})^2/\text{expected count}$$

TABLE 7.3
Leprosin A skin tests in various subject groups

	Test result		
	Positive	Negative	Total
Healthy controls (A)	30	20	50
Hospital contacts (B)	18	2	20
Household contacts (C)	45	33	78
Treated patients (D)	35	18	53
New (untreated) patients (E)	21	31	52
Total	149	104	253

MTB > NAME C1 'POS.'
MTB > NAME C2 'NEG.'
MTB > CHISQ C1 C2

Expected counts are printed below observed counts

	POS.	NEG.	Total
1	30	20	50
	29·45	20·55	
2	18	2	20
	11·78	8·22	
3	45	33	78
	45·94	32·06	
4	35	18	53
	31·21	21·79	
5	21	31	52
	30·62	21·38	
Total	149	104	253

ChiSq = 0·010 + 0·015 +
        3·286 + 4·708 +
        0·019 + 0·027 +
        0·459 + 0·658 +
        3·025 + 4·334 = 16·541
df = 4

MTB > CDF 16·541;
SUBC> CHISQ 4.
    16·5410   0·9976

NOTE: so the p value of the test is $1 - 0.9976 = 0.0024$.

Figure 7.6   Minitab output for the χ^2 analysis of the Leprosin A skin test data (table 7.3). The highly significant χ^2 value indicates that some of the groups differ in responsiveness.

for all 10 cells of the table giving the value of 16·54, which has a P value of 0·0024. This indicates that the data provide extremely strong evidence of differences between some of the population proportions. To follow up this finding we can calculate a series of multiple confidence intervals for the difference between positive response rates. The details of this procedure are given in the Appendix. Confidence intervals for the differences between positive response rates for each pair of groups are displayed in fig 7.7, from which it is apparent that the main difference is between hospital contacts of patients with leprosy who have the highest rate of positive response and the group of new patients who have the

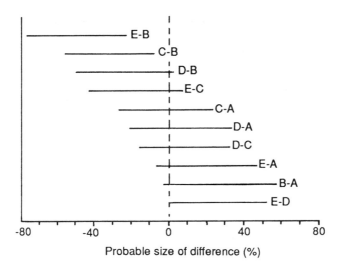

Figure 7.7 Multiple comparison confidence intervals for the differences between proportions of positive skin tests for all pairs of groups of subjects. Most of the intervals include zero, indicating that the corresponding pair of groups cannot be regarded as differing in responsiveness. To indicate the groups being compared the lines representing the confidence intervals are labelled with letters assigned to the groups in table 7.3.

lowest positive response rate. The remaining groups fall in an intermediate position and there are no detectable differences between their response rates.

Multiple category responses

The χ^2 test may also be applied to situations where there are more than two categories of response. Table 7.4 shows the results of an

TABLE 7.4
Relation between BCG vaccination status and cavitation of lung in Indonesian patients with pulmonary tuberculosis

Extent of cavitation	Vaccinated	Not vaccinated	Total
0	4	31	35
1	4	9	13
2	13	18	31
3	3	27	30
Total	24	85	109

investigation of the relation between BCG vaccination status and extent of cavitation of the lungs (graded on a four point ordinal scale) in Indonesian patients with pulmonary tuberculosis. The hypothesis that the underlying distribution of the extent of cavitation does not depend on the vaccination status of the patients is tested by the χ^2 method. A significant result will mean that extent of cavitation does depend on vaccination status. Expected values and the χ^2 statistic are calculated in the same way as in the previous examples and the Minitab output (fig 7.8A) indicates a problem with small sample sizes as one expected count is considerably less than 5. This may be dealt with by combining the first two cavitation categories (cavitation index none or one) to obtain higher expected counts. This leads to the analysis shown in fig 7.8B, from which we conclude that extent of cavitation is not independent of BCG vaccination status. The main difference between the distributions of extent of cavitation seems to be a relative excess of cavitation grade 2 (cavities in two lung zones) among the BCG vaccinated patients. Interpretation of this type of investigation is necessarily more complex as you are looking for differences in the overall pattern of the multiple category grading variable and such differences cannot be summarised in terms of one or two simply interpretable numbers.

Point or structure counts, radioactive counts

Where an investigation entails direct counts of structures in tissue sections or estimation of proportionate areas or volumes occupied by various features then although the end result will be expressed as a proportion, the method of analysis to be used is quite different from that described in the earlier sections of this chapter. The same will be true of investigations which use radioactive cpm as an indirect method of measuring some aspect of cellular activity, such as DNA synthesis. The essential difference is that each case will result in a separate proportion or count rather than contributing a small amount. In this case proportions and cpm can be treated as if they were measurements and all of the methods appropriate to measured data may be used after suitable transformation of the data.

Proportions and cpm, however, are not true measurements and they do not conform to all the assumptions that the standard methods devised for continuous data require for their validity. In

```
MTB > CHISQ C1 C2
         Expected counts are printed below observed counts
                    C1          C2          Total
    1               4           31          35
                    7·71        27·29

    2               4           9           13
                    2·86        10·14

    3               13          18          31
                    6·83        24·17

    4               3           27          30
                    6·61        23·39


 Total              24          85          109

ChiSq = 1·783 + 0·503 +
        0·452 + 0·128 +
        5·585 + 1·577 +
        1·968 + 0·556 = 12·551
df = 3
1 cells with expected counts less than 5·0
```

```
MTB > CHISQ C1 C2

         Expected counts are printed below observed counts
                    C1          C2          Total
    1               8           40          48
                    10·57       37·43

    2               13          18          31
                    6·83        24·17

    3               3           27          30
                    6·61        23·39

 Total              24          85          109

ChiSq = 0·624 + 0·176 +
        5·585 + 1·577 +
        1·968 + 0·556 = 10·486
df = 2
MTB > CDF 10·486;
SUBC> CHISQ 2.
   10·4860      0·9947

NOTE: So the p value of the test is 1 − 0·9947 = 0·0053.
```

Figure 7.8 (A) Minitab output for the data relating extent of lung cavitation to BCG vaccination status (table 7.4). One of the expected counts is less than 5, so the χ^2 test could be misleading. (B) By combining results for adjacent cavitation grades (0,1) the expected counts are raised to permit valid use of the χ^2 test.

particular, the assumption of constant residual variability is not met. The variability in a set of proportions is related to the size of the proportions, thus small and large proportions have less scope for being variable because they cannot extend beyond zero or unity, whereas the intermediate proportions have more room for variability. To nullify this effect proportions should, in this situation, always be transformed by means of the angular transformation[3] (also known as the arc-sine transformation) before methods such as analysis of variance or regression analysis are applied.

From the theory of radiation physics it can be shown that radioactive counts conform to the Poisson distribution, not the normal distribution. One of the important consequences of this is that the variability of radioactive cpm will be directly proportional to their average. In this situation the raw data must be transformed by taking square roots of counts before applying analysis of variance or regression methods.

Appendix

Expected counts and degrees of freedom
There is a simple rule for calculating the expected counts for each cell of the table:

$$\text{expected count} = \text{row total} \times \text{column total}/\text{grand total}.$$

The degrees of freedom associated with the χ^2 statistic are equal to one less than the number of rows in the table multiplied by one less than the number of columns.

Confidence intervals
The standard error of the estimate (p) of a proportion is $\sqrt{(p(1-p)/n)}$ and the confidence interval is:

$$\text{estimate} \pm \text{critical value} \times \text{SE of estimate}$$

The critical value is 1·96 for a 95% interval, 2·58 for a 99% interval, and 2·81 for a 99·5% interval. These critical values are the upper 2·5%, 0·5%, and 0·25% points of the normal distribution.

If the estimates of two proportions are p_1 and p_2 based on samples of sizes n_1 and n_2 then the standard error of their difference is:

$$\sqrt{(p_1(1-p_1)/n_1 + p_2(1-p_2)/n_2)}$$

and a confidence interval for the difference between the proportions is:

$$(p_1 - p_2) \pm \text{critical value} \times \text{SE of difference,}$$

the same critical values being used.

Multiple comparison of a set of proportions

The confidence intervals shown in fig 7.7 were calculated by applying the formula for the confidence interval for the difference between two proportions to all possible pairs of proportions. To maintain an overall error rate of 5% in the complete set of comparisons the confidence coefficient of each interval must be $100\% - 5\%/(\text{number of comparisons})$. In the example there are 10 comparisons so the confidence coefficient must be 99.5% and each interval will be of the form:

$$\text{difference} \pm 2.81 \times \text{SE of difference.}$$

For example, the proportion of positive skin tests among the hospital controls is 0.9 and among the healthy controls it is 0.6. The difference is 0.3 with a standard error equal to $\sqrt{(0.6 \times 0.4/50) + (0.9 \times 0.1/20))}$, or 0.096 so the confidence interval is $0.3 \pm 2.81 \times 0.096$ or 0.3 ± 0.27, $(30\% \pm 27\%)$. Note that a separate calculation of the standard error is needed for each pair of groups being compared.

Fisher's exact text

The exact test calculates the P value associated with the observed table on the hypothesis that there is no difference between the corresponding population proportions. This is done by summing the probability of occurrence of the observed table and all tables which have the same marginal totals but are more extreme than it is. In the example these are the tables shown in fig 7.9, which are obtained by putting 0, 1 and 2 in the upper top left corner. This then determines the remaining three entries because the row and column totals are fixed.

If O_1, O_2, O_3, and O_4 denotes the values in the body of the table, R_1, R_2, C_1, C_2, and N the row totals, column totals, and grand total,

0	7	7	1	6	7	2	5	7
9	4	13	8	5	13	7	6	13
9	11	20	9	11	20	9	11	20

Figure 7.9   The P value of Fisher's exact test is calculated by summing the probabilities of occurrence associated with these three tables (derived from table 7.2).

respectively, then the probability associated with this particular table is:

$$\frac{R_1! \times R_2! \times C_1! \times C_2!}{N! \times O_1! \times O_2! \times O_3! \times O_4!}$$

where, for example $R_1!$ (read as "R_1 factorial") is the product of the integers from 1 up to R_1, (in this example $R_1 = 7$ and $7! = 7 \times 6 \times 5 \times 4 \times 3 \times 2 \times 1$ or 5040). Note also that the numerical value of 0! (zero factorial) is 1.

The probabilities associated with the three tables in fig 7.9 are

$(7! \times 13! \times 9! \times 11!)/(20! \times 7! \times 9! \times 4!)$,
$(7! \times 13! \times 9! \times 11!)/(20! \times 1! \times 6! \times 8! \times 5!)$ and
$(7! \times 13! \times 9! \times 11!)/(20! \times 2! \times 5! \times 7! \times 6!)$ or 0·004, 0·053, and 0·215,

so the P value of the observed table is 0·272, leading to the conclusion that observed results provide no evidence of a difference between the proportions.

8

Statistical methods for diagnostic tests

Reference ranges

Most tests used in clinical medicine give a numerical result on a continuous measurement scale. The pathologists or clinicians attempt to interpret the result by comparing it with a "reference range" previously calculated from a study of people who do not have the disease in question. By current convention, the reference range includes all but the top and bottom 2·5% of the results expected from a population of healthy people, so that 5% of the "normal" healthy population will have test values falling outside the reference range. Consequently, the fact that the test result for an individual subject is outside the reference range does not necessarily imply that the individual is abnormal—this is one reason why the older term "normal range" is becoming obsolete.

A reference range may be determined from test values obtained from a sample of healthy subjects, provided (i) the subjects constitute a random sample from the healthy portion of the population and (ii) the sample size is sufficiently large for it to be representative of the population and for the sample mean and standard deviation to be precise estimates of the population mean and standard deviation.

If the population distribution of the test results is normal, then 95% of all values will lie within the range:

population mean ± 1.96 (population standard deviation)

(chapter 2). The sample mean and standard deviation are estimates of the unknown population mean and standard deviation and by convention the *reference range* is taken to be:

sample mean ± 1.96 (sample standard deviation)

The sample mean and standard deviation are, however, subject to sampling variation—that is, each random sample gives rise to different sample statistics—and so the limits of the reference range will be imprecise. Confidence intervals can be calculated for the upper and lower reference limits to indicate the imprecision of the reference range. If the sample size is large a 95% confidence interval for each end of the reference range is:

$$\text{reference limit} \pm 1 \cdot 96 \sqrt{3} \text{ (SE mean)}.$$

The method for calculation can be illustrated by data obtained in a study of the prevalence and titre of IgE antibodies to *Mycobacterium tuberculosis* in healthy Indonesian factory workers (group A, fig 8.1). The distribution of the counts in the radioallergosorbent test (RAST) is not symmetrical but it becomes so after logarithmic transformation. These log-transformed results have a reference range of 1·42 to 3·20; the 95% confidence interval calculation indicates that the upper limit for the upper end of the range is 3·28 and the lower limit for the lower end point is 1·34. If these limits are back-transformed (using antilogs) this results in a reference range of 22 to 1905 cpm.

The concept of a reference range is not restricted to medical diagnosis but appears in the guise of a "tolerance interval" in industrial quality control. Comprehensive information on the internationally accepted definition of a statistical tolerance interval is contained in ISO Standard 3207.[17] The validity of the calculations of the reference range and the confidence intervals for the reference limits depends very critically on the assumption that the test values are normally distributed, so the sample must be assessed for normality and possible outliers using methods described in chapter 2 before starting the reference range calculation. If the data are not normally distributed or contain inexplicable outliers the sample mean and standard deviation method cannot be used to determine the reference range. If the data are skewed to the right, a square root or a logarithmic transformation (as used with the data of fig 8.1) may bring about symmetry and perhaps normality, thus allowing calculation by the above method.

Usually it will be safer to determine reference limits by a method which does not require normality of the raw test results. A universally applicable method is based on the percentiles of the observed distribution of the sample values. Any given percentile is

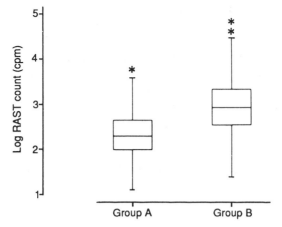

Figure 8.1 Box and whisker plots comparing titre of IgE antibodies to Mycobacterium tuberculosis using the radioallergosorbent test (RAST) in 350 healthy Indonesian factory workers (group A) and 350 Indonesian tuberculosis patients (group B). Both distributions are symmetrical on a logarithmic scale.
Group A: mean of log counts = 2·31, SD of log counts = 0·45.
Group B: mean of log counts = 2·96, SD of log counts = 0·58.

that value below which a specified percentage of the distribution lies; so 2·5% of the sample values do not exceed the 2·5 percentile and 97·5% of sample values do not exceed the 97·5 percentile (this is analogous to the quartiles introduced in chapter 2). On condition that the sample size is sufficiently large, this provides a very simple method of determining reference limits. Statgraphics will automatically calculate any specified percentiles of a set of results and for the test results of the healthy workers shown in fig 8.1 the 2·5 and 97·5 percentiles of the untransformed RAST counts are 26 and 1518. This technique will only produce reliable results if the sample size is sufficiently large for the sample to be representative of the variability in the population (greater than 100 to be safe). For small samples the sample percentiles will be very imprecise estimates of the corresponding population values. A 95% confidence interval for the 2·5 percentile may be found as follows: first calculate,

$$0.025 \text{ (sample size)} \pm 1.96 \sqrt{(0.025 \times 0.975 \times \text{sample size})}$$

This will give two values which will not usually be integers: then round the values up to the next integer.[18] For example, if the

89

sample size is 350 then the above calculation gives the values 3·48 and 14·02 which are rounded up to 4 and 15. This means that the 95% confidence interval for the 2·5 percentile stretches from the 4th smallest up to the 15th smallest test value (17 to 32). The corresponding interval for the 97·5 percentile is determined by counting down the same number of values from the largest test value (giving 1180 to 1995). Thus the reference range based on percentiles, and allowing for uncertainty in the percentiles, is 17 to 1995, which is not very different from that found by using the previous method based on the assumption of normality of log RAST count.

There are several sources of variation which are likely to affect the test value produced by any well monitored and accurately calibrated analytical technique for a given subject. For example (a) inherent random error in the analysis of the sample, usually monitored by quality control methods, (b) time-related variation, (c) variation associated with physiological changes, (d) variation associated with external factors such as diet, tobacco, or alcohol consumption, exercise, posture, and so on, before taking the test specimen. Such factors will tend to increase the variability of results and, in the absence of information about the magnitude of their effects on variability it may be difficult to interpret a result which lies "just outside" the reference range. Thus a healthy subject who has a "true" value close to the upper reference limit may give a test result above the limit. Similarly, a diseased subject who has a "true" value above the upper reference limit could be within the reference range when tested.

Assessment of diagnostic tests

In view of the uncertainties inherent in comparing a test result with a reference range it is worth while examining the criteria that should be used in assessing and choosing diagnostic tests.[19 20] To assess a particular diagnostic method results must first be obtained from a group of subjects who have the fully developed disease and a group in which the disease is absent. In practice, diagnostic tests are often used to assess patients who are in the early stages of disease; this raises the issue of whether comparison of the above groups addresses the correct question. The criteria for determining the presence and absence of the disease in these two groups must be carefully stated and should agree with standard well understood and accepted methodology (a "gold" standard). The criteria for what constitutes a positive test result must be carefully and unambiguously stated. For example, if the test result is determined by comparison of peaks on a chart then the precise way in which the peaks are located and exactly how they are compared should be explained unambiguously.

If the initial studies on a proposed new diagnostic method were based on 350 healthy subjects and 350 patients with pulmonary tuberculosis patients who have been diagnosed as having the disease on the basis of some independent, well defined, and accepted criterion (in this case chext x ray pictures), the test results might be as shown in fig 8.1. The investigator might perform a Mann-Whitney test (chapter 5), as the test results are not normally distributed, the resulting P value being less than 0·0001.

The investigator would be wrong to conclude from this that the assay has high diagnostic value because the Mann-Whitney test is designed to answer the question, "do the data provide evidence of a difference in the medians of the population distributions for healthy and diseased persons?" This is largely irrelevant for judging the clinical value of a diagnostic test, where the critical decision *must* involve a notion of a cut off point to assist in decision taking. In practice, values above a certain critical limit will be regarded as indicating that the patient has the disease and lower values that it is unlikely that the patient has the disease. The pertinent question must concern not merely the separation between the medians (or means) of the corresponding population distributions for the healthy and diseased groups but separation of the distributions *as a whole*. It is relatively common for the distributions to overlap (fig 3.1), and this raises the possibility that a healthy subject will be classified as diseased or that a diseased subject may be classified as healthy. Assessment of a diagnostic test must concentrate on such issues and look at the risks of misclassification.

As the initial assessment of the value of the proposed new test depends on its application to a group of patients with clearly established disease and to people who are undoubtedly healthy the results for any selected cut off point can be summarised in a 2×2 table as shown in fig 8.2. The *sensitivity* of a test is defined as the proportion of the patients who have the disease in whom the test result is positive ($a/(a + c)$), and this is a measure of the probability that a person who has the disease will give a positive test result.

		Disease Present	Absent	Total
Test result	Positive	a	b	a+b
	Negative	c	d	c+d
Total		a+c	b+d	a+b+c+d

Figure 8.2   For any specified cut off point the results of a single test on a group of patients with the disease and a group of controls without the disease may be classified into a 2 × 2 table.

The *specificity* of a test is defined as the proportion of healthy subjects in whom the test result is negative, $(d/(b+d))$, and this measures the probability that a healthy person will give a negative test result. The *false positive rate* is the proportion of healthy subjects who give a positive test result $(b/(b+d))$, and the *false negative rate* is the proportion of subjects who have the disease but give a negative result $(c/(a+c))$. Thus in this example with the cut off point set at an RAST count of 320 the test correctly identified 71·4% of those with the disease, but failed to detect the disease in 28·6% of cases. It also correctly identified 72·6% of those who were disease free but was positive in 27·4% of cases where the disease was absent (fig 8.3).

Very few diagnostic tests have 100% sensitivity and 100% specificity and consequently it should be realised that although knowledge of these operating characteristics of a test are very important, this is not in itself sufficient to determine the probability that the disease is present when the test result is positive, or of absence when the test proves negative.

When selecting a test it is necessary to compare the sensitivity and specificity of the available tests. As a general rule, the test with

		Disease Present	Absent	Total
Test result	Positive	250	96	346
	Negative	100	254	354
Total		350	350	700

Figure 8.3   The observed incidence of positive and negative test results based on the data of figure 8.1 when a positive result is defined as a RAST count exceeding 320 cpm.

the highest sensitivity should be selected for clinical diagnosis unless its specificity is unacceptably low. When a test is to be applied for screening purposes it can be argued that it is important that as large a proportion as possible of those who give a positive test result do, in fact, have the disease the screening program is meant to detect, and so the sensitivity should be high. A test used to confirm a diagnosis should have a high specificity—that is, it should produce a negative result in a high proportion of those who do not have the disease.

The sensitivity and specificity of a test can be changed by altering the criterion for positivity. When the test gives numerical values on a continuous scale a cut off point is used to define the boundary between positive and negative results—for example, in fig 8.1 a cut off point at 500 (log 500 = 2·699) results in a sensitivity of 66% and a specificity of 77%. By moving the cut off point down the scale a greater proportion of diseased subjects will give a positive test result so the sensitivity increases, but this occurs at the cost of fewer subjects without the disease giving a negative result— that is, decreasing specificity. The *receiver–operator characteristic* *(ROC) curve* of a test is a graph which is constructed by plotting, for a series of cut off points, the sensitivity (true positive rate) against the false positive rate (100-specificity). This curve is shown in fig 8.4 for the data displayed in fig 8.1, and it is apparent that the test cannot provide a very high true positive rate coupled with a

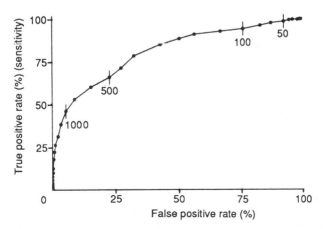

Figure 8.4 Receiver-operator characteristic curve (ROC) for a hypothetical diagnostic test based on the RAST counts of figure 8.1. Selected cut off points are marked.

93

low false positive rate. The ROC may be used to determine the optimal cut off point for the test according to the costs and benefits (in the widest sense) resulting from correct and incorrect diagnoses. Competing tests may be assessed by comparing their ROC curves.

The probability that a patient with a positive test result has the disease depends not only on the sensitivity and specificity of the test but also on the pre-test or prior estimate of the probability that a patient presenting with a particular combination of signs and symptoms has the disease. Note that an investigation designed to assess a test and determine its ROC curve does not provide this information because the assessment will be based on approximately equal numbers of healthy and diseased subjects. The prior estimate of disease probability must be based on past experience of the prevalence of the disease among patients with the specified signs and symptoms.

If the prior estimate was—for example, 50%—that is, in 2000 patients presenting 1000 would be expected to have the disease—then the data from the test evaluation may be combined with this information to give the results shown in fig 8.5. Of the 1000 patients with the disease, 714 will give a positive test result and 274 of the 1000 patients who do not have the disease will also be positive. Consequently, 988 positive test results would be expected, and the proportion of diseased patients among these is 714 out of 988 or 72·3%. Thus a positive test result converts a 50% chance that the patient has the disease into a 72% chance. The *positive predictive value* (PPV) of a positive rest result is the probability that a patient who gives a positive test has the disease and the *predictive value of a negative result* (PVN) is the corresponding probability that a patient with a negative result does not

| | | Disease | | Total |
		Present	Absent	
Test	Positive	714	274	988
result	Negative	286	726	1022
	Total	1000	1000	2000

Figure 8.5 Expected numbers of subjects in the four categories in a group of 2000 subjects if a positive test result is defined as a RAST count exceeding 320 cpm, when the prior estimate of the disease probability is 0·5.

TABLE 8.1

Prior estimate of disease probability	Positive predictive value	Predictive value of a negative result
0·1	0·225	0·958
0·3	0·528	0·856
0·5	0·723	0·717
0·7	0·859	0·521
0·9	0·959	0·220

have the disease. Table 8.1 shows the positive and negative predictive value for prior estimates ranging from 10% to 90% when the sensitivity and specificity of the test are 71·4% and 72·6%. In this case the results are not particularly impressive, which is a reflection of the fact that the RAST count is not a good diagnostic indicator in this particular situation.

It must be borne in mind that the results of an assessment of a diagnostic test, which compares those without the disease and those with fully developed disease, are likely to overstate the predictive value of a positive or a negative result when the test is applied to patients who do not have the fully developed disease because the distribution of test results in such patients is likely to be closer to that of the disease free group than the distribution of test results from patients with fully developed disease.

Discriminant analysis

There are many clinical situations in which a single diagnostic test may not be sufficiently specific or sensitive to diagnose a disease and it is usual to perform two or more different tests and base the diagnosis on the combined results. The assessment of such situations leads naturally to investigation of the sensitivity and specificity of the combination of two or more tests. *Discriminant analysis* is the method generally chosen for determining objectively the cut off region between controls and patients. For example, assays for serum factor VIII based on radioimmunoassay and bioassay were compared for their diagnostic value in detecting women who were carriers of haemophilia.[21] The results for each test taken separately showed substantial overlap between women who were carriers and controls. When, however, the results were displayed in a scatter-plot, it was clear that the two groups could be separated almost

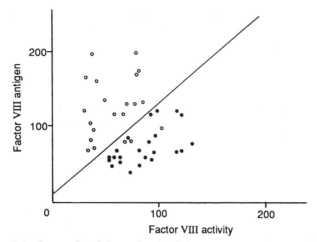

Figure 8.6   Scatterplot of the results of radioimmunoassay (antigen) and bioassay (activity) of serum factor VIII in 21 definite female carriers of haemophilia (○) and 23 normal women (●). The straight line indicates the linear discriminant function.

completely by an imaginary diagonal line (fig 8.6). On this basis it would be possible to set out the rule, "classify the subject as a carrier if the results of the pair of tests lie above the line." For this cut off line the sensitivity is 86% and the specificity is 100%, so the combination of the two tests is an immense improvement over the use of either test alone.

Discriminant analysis[22][23] is the name given to the statistical technique for determining objectively the position of the line which best discriminates between the two groups, in the sense of producing as few misclassifications as possible in the data from the original investigation. The line separating the two groups defines the *linear discriminant function* which is merely a formula for combining both test results into a single *discriminant score* which may then be used to assess sensitivity and specificity in the usual way. The Statgraphics output for the data of fig 8.6 is shown in fig 8.7, the "unstandardised discriminant function coefficients" are interpreted in the following way: for each of the 44 women calculate:

$$0{\cdot}0347 \text{ (factor VIII activity)} - 0{\cdot}0272 \text{(factor VIII antigen)} + 0{\cdot}2853,$$

Discriminant analysis for factor VIII	
Unstandardised discriminant function coefficients	
	1
Activity	0·0347
Antigen	−0·0272
CONSTANT	0·2853

Figure 8.7   Statgraphics output for linear discriminant analysis of the data of figure 8.6.

this is the discriminant score for each woman. Whether a person is classified by *the data alone* as a carrier or as normal depends on whether her score is positive or negative; negative scores are indicative of carrier status. Obviously, anyone with a zero score cannot be classified and this fact allows the discriminating line to be drawn. We may rewrite this condition as discriminant score = 0 or as:

$$0·0272(\text{factor VIII antigen}) = 0·0347(\text{factor VIII activity}) + 0·2853,$$

On dividing throughout by 0·0272 this becomes:

$$\text{factor VIII antigen} = 1·28(\text{factor VIII activity}) + 10·50,$$

which is the equation of the straight line drawn in fig 8.6. The discriminant score for any subject is related to the perpendicular distance from this line to the point corresponding to her activity and antigen results.

The discrimination is not perfect; three of the known carriers are misclassified as normal. The overall misclassification rate of 3 out of 21 carriers and 0 out of 23 normal controls is bound to be somewhat overoptimistic as an estimate of what is likely to happen if the rule is used in future, because the discriminant function is designed to minimise the total proportion of those who are misclassified for the available data. The discriminant scores for both groups are plotted in fig 8.8 and show almost complete separation of the groups.

The sensitivity and specificity of the pair of tests may be examined by calculating the misclassification rates for other cut off

97

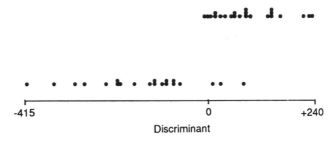

Figure 8.8   Plot of the discrimination scores for the data of figure 8.6.

points than that resulting from the discriminant analysis. This is done by replacing the constant in the discriminant score (0·2853) by a range of alternatives. The data manipulation facilities of Statgraphics can be used to calculate the discriminant score 0·0347(factor VIII activity) − 0·0272(factor VII antigen) for each person in both the control and the carrier group and the tabulation facilities can be used to calculate how many subjects of either group have a discriminant score less than each alternative cut off value, and from this the sensitivity and specificity at each alternative value can be determined which enables the ROC curve to be plotted.

Discriminant analysis is not limited to pairs of measurements, it may be applied to situations where several different measurements have been made on each of several subjects in different groups with the intention of finding linear discriminant functions which allow newly observed subjects to be allocated to one of the groups. It should be noted, however, that the method will be reliable only if the subjects used in the original investigation were allocated to the groups by some well understood and reliable method.

The method of discriminant analysis used by Statgraphics and similar packages cannot cope successfully with data which consist of a mixture of measurements (continuous variables) and categorical or ordinal data. Advice from your local statistical guru should be sought if your data include both types of variables.

9

Survival analysis

Some features of survival data

Medical research into methods of treating fatal conditions generally involves either an assessment of whether improved survival is associated with a particular treatment regimen, or it may attempt to determine whether patients with a greater chance of survival can be distinguished from those with a lesser chance on the basis of measurable features of the disease.

Survival analysis consists of a body of statistical techniques that can be used to quantify survival experience in a systematic way and to compare survival experience in different groups of patients, or to assess the relationship between survival time and other measured variables.

The fundamental measurement in any survival study is the *survival time*, which is defined as the time from some unambiguously defined starting point, (for example, the date of entry of the patient into the study, or the time at which diagnosis was made), until death. It might be argued that the true survival times of patients ought to be defined as the length of time from the start of their illness, but it is virtually impossible to determine this for all conditions of relatively gradual onset. A characteristic feature of survival data is that they tend to show high variability and marked asymmetry in their distribution.

Survival analysis methods are not restricted to the analysis of data obtained from a situation where the death of the patient is the end point, they are also applicable in other situations—for example, survival time could be the time until recurrence of a disease in patients who have undergone remission, or it could be the length of time before a hip joint replacement prosthesis begins to malfunction, although in this latter case "malfunction" would need to be defined carefully and unambiguously.

A typical well planned survival study must be quite a longterm affair: five to ten or more years would be quite common. If the condition is one where normal experience points to considerable variability in survival times, with some patients likely to survive for several years, then the study will need to extend over a long enough period of time to give worthwhile information about the chances of relatively longterm survival.

With the exception of newly recognised diseases such as AIDS, the pattern of survival for the commonly occurring diseases is fairly well quantified and so survival studies are not used simply to accumulate information about the chances of survival for various lengths of time. Survival studies are therefore designed, in the main, to make comparisons between survival experience for different treatment regimens, with the intention of determining whether any particular regimen enhances the prospects of survival. For convenience we will refer to this approach as a *comparison study*. Alternatively, survival times may be recorded along with other information which is suspected to be associated with length of survival and so may be of value in predicting survival time. For example, it might be conjectured that the length of survival for patients with a particular form of cancer could be related to (a) the size of the tumour, (b) aggressiveness of the disease expressed in some quantitative way such as extent of lymph node involvement, and (c) the age of the patient at diagnosis. The question that then springs to mind is whether it is possible to combine (a), (b), and (c) into some form of prognostic index. This would make a useful contribution to predicting any particular new patient's survival prospects, given his or her age, the size of their tumour, the aggressiveness value. This approach we will call a *prognostic study*.

Survival studies may be of two types, prospective and retrospective. Although a prospective study is preferable, since the investigator is in complete control of the planning and data collection, many studies are retrospective and so are somewhat less carefully designed and more opportunistic than one would wish.

Whatever its purpose, a typical prospective survival study will begin with a recruitment phase, when patients are entered into the study, and allocated to the relevant treatment regimen, taking care to follow a well defined protocol for deciding the eligibility of patients and for their allocation to treatment. After this will come the follow up phase, during which a proportion of the patients will die. At the end of the follow up phase the study is concluded and typically there will be a proportion of patients who are still alive at this point. The ideal would be to follow up every patient who

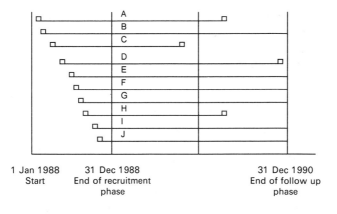

Figure 9.1   A hypothetical study in which ten patients are recruited, four die during the study period, and six are still alive at the end of the follow up period.

entered the study until death, but the need to collect results within a definite time and the constraints on the resources available for follow up often make this totally impractical. The lengths of the recruitment and follow up phases will be dependent on a number of factors.

All survival studies have to recruit a sufficiently large number of patients to provide some reasonable degree of confidence that it will be possible (a) to detect any clinically worthwhile difference in survival experience between treatment regimens in a comparison study, or (b) to construct a prognostic index which makes a medically worthwhile contribution to the clinician's judgment of survival prospects, in the case of a prognostic study. This has implications for the lengths of both phases of any survival study. The recruitment phase must be long enough to ensure that enough patients enter the study; and the follow up phase has to be long enough to provide meaningful data on survival times.

To appreciate how this introduces a complication which has not been encountered in any of the methods of data analysis treated in previous chapters, consider a hypothetical situation where 50% of patients may be expected to die within three years of diagnosis and suppose that a study is proposed which has a one year recruitment phase and a two year follow up phase. Clearly it would be expected that about 50% of patients will still be alive at the close, perhaps more if you allow for those who entered near the end of the recruitment phase. This is illustrated in fig 9.1, in which ten

101

patients are recruited during the first year, four die during the study, and six are alive at the close. The patients who are still alive at the end of the follow up phase cause something of a problem so far as the analysis of the data is concerned because the only information the investigator will have on these patients is the length of time they had survived up to the time the study was concluded. For example, the second patient entered the study on 1 March 1988, and was still alive at the close on 31 December 1990. This means that the most that can be said about this patient's survival time is that it is at least 34 months (or 1036 days).

Note that this is not the same as saying that this patient's survival time *is* 34 months. In fact, such an interpretation of the finding would be very misleading since the patient could live for some considerable time after the end of the study. When this occurs the survival times of those patients who are still alive at the close of the follow up phase are referred to as *censored* survival times. Patients who die during the study contribute *uncensored* survival times. Censoring can occur in most survival studies and it introduces complications into the data analysis.

The implication of this for the planning of the study is that the follow up phase should be long enough both to allow the estimation of the proportion of survivors over periods of time of particular interest and to ensure that censored survival times do not make up the bulk of the data. This suggests that it would be prudent to review very carefully the available information on survival experience as a prelude to the planning of a survival study. For example, in the hypothetical study outlined above it is clearly impossible to derive any meaningful information about the proportion of patients who survive for much more than 48 months because the total length of the study is so short. If you wished to compare the chances of survival for 48 months or longer under alternative treatment regimens the study would have to be at least four years in length, preferably with the follow up phase being at least four years long. Otherwise you would be taking a gamble on the actual recruitment pattern resulting in enough patients surviving for at least 48 months to make estimation of the underlying 48 month proportion reasonably precise.

Standard elementary methods of summarising and analysing data are not valid for survival data which includes censored survival times. For example, suppose you wished to summarise survival experience, it would be quite improper to calculate the mean survival time because the censored and uncensored survival times contribute different types of information. Someone who dies during a study 22 months after diagnosis has a survival time of 22 months, but someone who is diagnosed 28 months before the close of a study and is still alive at the close contributes the information only that their survival time is *at least* 28 months. Clearly the mean survival time cannot be calculated when the data are a mixture of censored and uncensored values as there is no way of handling "survived for at least 28 months," and it would be extremely misleading to treat the censored values as if they were uncensored, because the mean would then be an understatement of survival experience. As an alternative you might try to calculate the median survival time. This would be simple if you could be sure that all the censored survival times were in the upper tail of the distribution of observed censored and uncensored survival times. However, this may not be the case; some of the censored survival times could easily fall in the lower half of the distribution. You are then faced with the same problem as with the mean—ignoring the fact that they are censored values and giving them the ranks that their numerical values imply would give a biased result. For example, if the survival times in months of nine patients were:

$$27, 32, 41, 61, 63^*, 69^*, 70^*, 72^*, 82$$

where an asterisk denotes a censored survival time, it would not be valid to take the median survival time as 63 months. Suppose the four patients with censored times had been followed up until they died and they all turned out to have uncensored survival times greater than 82 months, which might easily happen; the median survival time would then be 82 months. This illustrates the difficulty of coping with censored data.

The survival curve

So far this discussion has referred in rather vague terms to "survival experience." It is now time to put the basic ideas of survival analysis on a more precise foundation. For most workers the ultimate aim for summarising survival data is to get the background knowledge to predict survival time for each individual patient. However, the factors governing survival are so diverse and

103

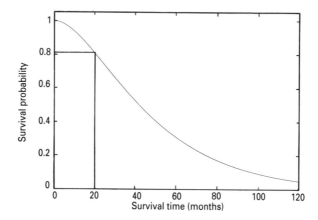

Figure 9.2 A typical population survival curve.

interact in such a complex way that it is just not possible to make predictions for specific individuals. Instead you have to be content with using statistical methods based on a sample of patients to estimate the probability of survival for a given length of time.

Theoretically, for each life threatening condition there is an underlying, but unobservable population survival distribution. Fig 9.2 is a graph of a typical survival distribution and it is possible to read off the chance that a randomly selected patient will have of surviving for at least a specified time. For instance, choosing 20 months and reading off the corresponding probability we see that in this case there is just over an 80% chance of surviving for at least 20 months, with the obvious corollary that there is just under a 20% chance of dying before 20 months have elapsed.

The population survival curve is acceptable as a theoretical foundation but it has practical difficulties: the analogy with the population distribution of a measurement and the histogram derived from values measured in a sample of patients, which underlies statistical methods for measured data, suggests that it is not a simple matter to obtain a precise picture of a survival curve. To achieve this it would be necessary to follow a very large number of patients through from diagnosis to death, and the sheer scale of such a study could cause great practical difficulties.

In reality most clinical survival studies have a restricted time span and involve a comparatively small number of patients. Such a study involving perhaps one or two hundred patients will only provide information from which an *estimate* of the underlying

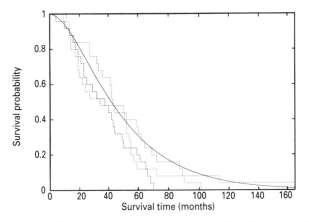

Figure 9.3   Comparison of empirical survival curves based on 25 subjects with the population survival curve.

survival curve known as the *empirical survival curve* can be obtained. This has two consequences: firstly, the empirical survival curve is not a smooth curve but looks more like a badly made staircase with treads of varying heights and widths, and secondly, allowance has to be made for sampling variability in interpreting or comparing survival curves. For instance, two survival studies of the same condition using identical protocols but recruiting different patients will not produce identical empirical survival curves, because the survival times of the patients are unlikely to be identical. This is illustrated in fig 9.3 where the smooth curve, which is the underlying population survival curve, is compared with the three "staircases" corresponding to estimated survival curves based on three hypothetical groups of 25 patients selected randomly from that population.

Another important factor is that a study of larger numbers of patients results in a more precise estimate of the survival curve. This is shown in fig 9.4: computer simulation was used to generate hypothetical survival times for progressively larger groups of patients. The discrepancies between the empirical survival curve and the underlying population survival curve become progressively smaller as the size of the group increases.

The Kaplan-Meier estimation method

The following simple arithmetical problem illustrates an important principle which is used in calculating survival probabilities. A

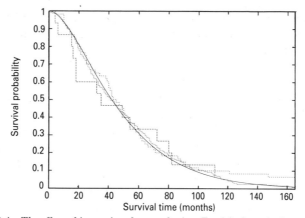

Figure 9.4   The effect of increasing the sample size. Empirical survival curves for sample of sizes 15, 60, and 240 compared with the population survival curve.

certain disease kills 10% of its victims per month: what percentage of an initial group of patients will still be alive after (a) one month, (b) two months, (c) five months? Clearly 90% of the group will still be alive after one month and they constitute the group at risk of death in the second month: the 10% who die in the second month amount to 9% of the original group so there will be 81% still alive after two months. After five months there will be

$$0{\cdot}9 \times 0{\cdot}9 \times 0{\cdot}9 \times 0{\cdot}9 \times 0{\cdot}9 \times 100\%$$

which is just over 59% of the original group still surviving.

This simple repetitive procedure applies whatever the proportion dying per month may be, for example if the percentages dying per month in each of the first five months were 10%, 12%, 15%, 30%, and 50% respectively, then after two months 79·2% would still be alive, after three months the figure would be 67·3%, after four months it would be 47·1%, and after five months only 23·6% of the original group would still be alive.

Having reviewed this basic principle we may now turn to the fundamental problem of constructing an estimated survival curve from a mixed set of uncensored and censored survival times by the Kaplan-Meier or "product limit" method. This is a non-parametric method which makes no assumptions whatsoever about the underlying survival distribution save that it takes the form of a

106

continuous curve. For simplicity of exposition the method will first be described for a sample which contains no censored times and no tied survival times.

First the survival times are ordered. Over the interval preceding the first death the estimated survival probability is given the value one. At the time corresponding to the first death the survival probability falls to a value equal to the proportion of those initially at risk who are still alive immediately after the time of the first death, and takes this value until the time of the second death. At this point it decreases once more to a value which is calculated by multiplying the survival probability in the first time interval by the proportion of patients at risk just after the first death who are still alive immediately after the time of the second death. From this point on the calculation is essentially a repetition of what has gone before. In the time interval between two successive deaths the survival probability is constant but decreases at the end of the interval to a value which is the product of its value in the interval in question and the proportion of those at risk during the interval who are still alive immediately after the end of the interval.

For example, if 50 patients were recruited into a study and the three shortest survival times were 6, 9, and 13 months then the survival probability would take the value $1 \cdot 0$ in the interval from 0 to 6 months, would fall to $^{49}/_{50}$ immediately after 6 months, and would remain at this value until 9 months, when it would fall to $^{49}/_{50} \times ^{48}/_{49}$ or $^{48}/_{50}$, remaining at this value until 13 months, when it would fall once again to $^{48}/_{50} \times ^{47}/_{48}$ or $^{47}/_{50}$. Note that in the particular case where all patients are followed up until death and there are no tied survival times the estimated survival probability decreases by

$$\frac{1}{\text{total number of patients}}$$

at the times at which individual deaths occur.

For the case where there are no censored survivals but some survival times are tied the same principle applies, except that the number of individuals surviving after a time corresponding to multiple deaths will be decreased by however many deaths occur at that time. Continuing with the previous example suppose that three deaths occurred after 6 months, two after 9 months, and four after 13 months, then the survival probability would be $1 \cdot 0$ until 6

107

months and would then fall to $^{47}/_{50}$. It would take this value until 9 months, when it would fall to $^{47}/_{50} \times ^{45}/_{47}$ or $^{45}/_{50}$ and remain at this value until 13 months when a further fall to $^{45}/_{50} \times ^{41}/_{45}$ or $^{41}/_{50}$ would take place.

The presence of censored survival times introduces a slight additional complication into the calculations: the survival probability still remains constant during the time interval between successive deaths, but censored survival times must be taken into account in determining the number at risk during that interval. The rule is that, when calculating the proportion of those at risk during the interval who are still alive immediately after the end of the interval, any individuals whose censored survival times fall within the interval in question must be deducted from the number at risk at the start of the interval. Finally, if censored survival times are tied with uncensored times the convention is that the ties are broken by assuming that the censored times are fractionally greater than the uncensored times. Of course, in principle there ought not to be any ties of either uncensored or censored times if all times were recorded sufficiently accurately, but in practice the smallest unit of time of interest may be a day, a week, or a month, and so on, may mean that all times are rounded to the nearest appropriate unit. While rounding to the nearest day is unlikely to cause serious distortion it does seem rather cavalier to round to the nearest month!

All of the details of handling ties and censored times are illustrated in the numerical calculation of the survival probabilities arising from a small retrospective study of patients from the breast clinic who have malignant cells in a pleural aspirate for which the survival times are given in table 9.1. The survival times have been ordered and an asterisk denotes a censored survival time.

The first event is a death after 9 months, when one of the original 20 patients dies, so the 9 month survival rate is 19/20 or 0·95. The subsequent calculations may be set out as shown in table 9.2. Only the times at which deaths occur need to be tabulated and the number at risk at any particular time is equal to the number of patients minus the number of deaths and the number of censored survivals which have occurred up to the time in question. Thus two patients die after 16 months and the number at risk just prior to this is 20 minus the two deaths after 9 and 12 months, minus the three censored survivals at 12, 13, and 14 months, giving 15 patients at risk.

TABLE 9.1
Survival times in months for patients from the breast
clinic who have malignant cells in a pleural aspirate.
Censored times are denoted by an asterisk.

Patient rank	Survival time (m)	Patient rank	Survival time (m)
1	9	11	27
2	12	12	29*
3	12*	13	30
4	13*	14	32
5	14*	15	33*
6	16	16	33*
7	16	17	34
8	19	18	35
9	23*	19	35
10	24*	20	36*

Automated calculation of the Kaplan-Meier estimate of a survival curve is available in the NANOSTAT package and was used to plot fig 9.5 which shows the survival curve for the data given in table 9.2. Other packages such as SPSS-PC and SAS also perform survival analysis. Minitab does not, although the ability of Minitab to obey a series of instructions known as a "macro" would enable the calculations to be done: this would need the assistance of your local statistician.

Comparing two or more survival curves

In a comparison study with patients allocated to different treatment regimens the question of interest is whether any treatment results in appreciably improved survival experience, or whether the data suggest that all treatments are equally (in)effective. The situation bears a superficial resemblance to those which would be analysed using the two sample t test or the analysis of variance, depending on the number of treatments being compared, but such methods would be totally inappropriate for analysis of survival for two reasons: firstly, survival data is invariably very highly non-normal in distribution, and secondly, the t test and similar analyses provide an assessment of differences between *population means*, whereas an analysis of survival data must be concerned with assessing the evidence for or against differences between *population*

TABLE 9.2
Calculation of the survival probabilities for the breast clinic survival data

Survival time	Number at risk	Number of deaths	Conditional survival rate	Unconditional survival rate
9	20	1	$\frac{19}{20}=0{\cdot}9500$	0·9500
12	19	1	$\frac{18}{19}=0{\cdot}9474$	0·9000
16	15	2	$\frac{13}{15}=0{\cdot}8667$	0·7801
19	13	1	$\frac{12}{13}=0{\cdot}9231$	0·7201
27	10	1	$\frac{9}{10}=0{\cdot}9000$	0·6481
30	8	1	$\frac{7}{8}=0{\cdot}8750$	0·5671
32	7	1	$\frac{6}{7}=0{\cdot}8571$	0·4860
34	4	1	$\frac{3}{4}=0{\cdot}7500$	0·3645
35	3	2	$\frac{1}{3}=0{\cdot}3333$	0·1215

survival time distributions, which is clearly a much more general question.

You should always start by drawing the empirical survival curves for the various groups of patients, and fig 9.6 shows these curves for data taken from a retrospective study of survival experience in two groups of patients with rectal carcinoma who were treated using two different radiotherapy regimens. The survival times for the two groups are given in table 9.3. Note that because the study was retrospective the sizes of the groups are different, and a number of patients in group B were at risk for rather a short time before the study end point. As a result there are rather more censored data in group B than would be ideal.

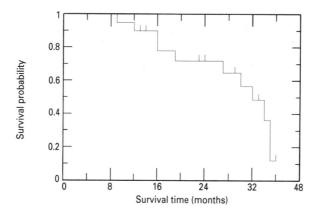

Figure 9.5   The survival curve produced by Nanostat for the data given in table 9.2.

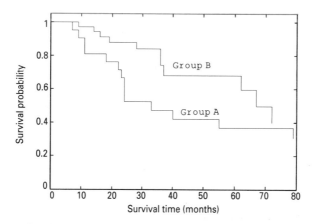

Figure 9.6   Survival curves for the two groups of patients with rectal cancer based on the data given in table 9.3.

The appropriate test is known as the Mantel-Haenszel test, after its inventors, but it is sometimes referred to as the log-rank test. The calculations for the test are in principle quite simple if rather tedious. First the results for both groups are combined and the time span of the study is divided into contiguous but non-overlapping time intervals, each one ending at a time which corresponds to a death. Often an interval will contain only one death but it could contain more, if several deaths occurred in one

111

TABLE 9.3.
Survival times of two groups of patients with rectal cancer treated with different radiotherapy regimens. An asterisk denotes a censored survival time.

Survival times (months)							
Group A			Group B				
7	24	71*	9	19	30*	36*	64*
9	24	79	14	24*	32*	36*	67
11	24	80*	14*	24*	34*	37	72
11	28*	83*	15*	26*	34*	39*	84*
18	33	92*	15*	26*	36	52*	89*
22	40	147*	16	28	36	55*	98*
23	55	148*	18*	29*	36*	62	130*

TABLE 9.4
Two way table classifying patients into those who die and those who survive within 11–14 months

	Deaths	Survivors	Total at risk
Group A	0	17	17
Group B	1	33	34
Total	1	50	51

or both groups after the same length of time at risk. The first few time intervals in this case are 0–7 months, 7–9 months, 9–11 months, and so on.

For each interval the number of deaths occurring in that interval and the number of patients who survive beyond the end of the interval looking at each group in turn can be set out in a two way table analogous to those used in analysing categorical data—in fact the classification of patients into those who die in the interval and those who survive has produced two categories. Table 9.4 shows this for the interval 11–14 months.

The expected number of deaths for each group, based on the assumption that there is no difference between the population survival distributions for the two populations of which the groups are supposed to be random samples, is calculated by dividing the total number of deaths by the total number at risk in the interval and then multiplying by the number at risk in the corresponding group (table 9.5).

TABLE 9.5
Two way table: total number of deaths divided by total number at risk within 11–14 months, multiplied by number at risk in corresponding group

	Deaths	Survivors	Total at risk
Group A	0·33	16·67	17
Group B	0·67	33·33	34
Total	1	50	51

TABLE 9.6
The calculation of expected deaths for the Mantel-Haenszel test.

Time	Total deaths	Total at risk	No. at risk in group A	Expected deaths in group A	No. at risk in group B	Expected deaths in group B
7	1	56	21	0·37500	35	0·62500
9	2	55	20	0·72727	35	1·27273
11	2	53	19	0·71698	34	1·28302
14	1	51	17	0·33333	34	0·66667
16	1	47	17	0·36170	30	0·63830
18	1	46	17	0·36957	29	0·63043
19	1	44	16	0·36364	28	0·63636
22	1	43	16	0·37209	27	0·62791
23	1	42	15	0·35714	27	0·64286
24	3	41	14	1·02439	27	1·97561
28	1	34	11	0·32353	23	0·67647
33	1	29	10	0·34483	19	0·65517
36	2	26	9	0·6923	17	1·307691
37	1	21	9	0·42857	12	0·57143
40	1	19	9	0·47368	10	0·52632
55	1	17	8	0·47059	9	0·52941
62	1	15	7	0·46667	8	0·53333
67	1	13	7	0·53846	6	0·46154
72	1	11	6	0·54545	5	0·45455
79	1	10	6	0·60000	4	0·40000
				9·8852		15·115

A similar calculation has then to be done for each interval (table 9.6). The result is an expected number of deaths for each group over the whole time span, obtained by summing the expected numbers of deaths over all intervals. The observed number of deaths in each group is then compared with the expected number using the familiar χ^2 statistic to make the comparison. Since 14

113

deaths occurred in group A and 11 in group B compared with expected values of 9·885 and 15·115 respectively

$$\chi^2 = \frac{(14 - 9\cdot885)^2}{9\cdot885} + \frac{(11 - 15\cdot115)^2}{15\cdot115}$$

or 2·86 with one degree of freedom. Large values of the χ^2 statistic are an indication that the underlying population distributions are different, and to assess the statistical significance of the value obtained here we must compare it with the percentage points of the χ^2 distribution with one degree of freedom. The P value corresponding to 2·86 is 0·091, so we conclude that the data provide rather weak evidence of a difference in the underlying survival distributions of populations represented by the individuals in the two groups.

Extending the method to more than two groups involves no new principles. The expected numbers of deaths in each group, assuming no difference between survival experience in any of the groups, would be calculated in a similar way to that shown in the example. The observed numbers of deaths would then be compared with the expected numbers by calculating a χ^2 statistic. This would be assessed for statistical significance by comparing it with the percentage points of the χ^2 distribution with degrees of freedom one less than the number of groups being compared, large values of the statistic indicating evidence against the hypothesis that the underlying survival distributions were the same for all groups. Of course the estimated survival curves should always be presented as a further aid to interpretation of the results of the statistical test.

Prognostic indicators and Cox regression

Prediction of survival for particular patients is fraught with difficulty since the factors governing length of survival of individuals are poorly understood. Nevertheless, groups of investigators have continued to attempt to relate survival to a range of variables which can be measured at diagnosis or during the course of treatment. The fundamental problem can be simply stated: find a set of measurements which are sufficiently well correlated with survival time that they can be used to give a reasonably reliable indicator of survival prospects. Studies which have attempted to do this have so far not been spectacularly successful. It may be more fruitful therefore to regard this area as one where investigations are largely exploratory in nature. In this case the problem is modified: given the survival times, censored and uncensored, of a number of patients, together with values for a number of clinical or physiological measurements which may be related to survival, determine those measurements, if any, which are so related and provide a numerical measure of how they are so related. This is suggestive of the general technique of regression analysis described in chapter 6, but because of the special nature of survival data new methods are required.

As a hypothetical example, an investigator might wish to relate survival time in breast cancer patients to age at diagnosis, size of tumour, and a measure of the aggressiveness of the tumour cells. The ultimate aim is to combine the three prognostic variables into a prognostic indicator of survival so that for any new patient the three values could be used to determine a survival curve. The technique which can be used to construct such an indicator and the corresponding survival curve is known as Cox regression, after its originator, Sir David Cox, but is also referred to as proportional hazards regression.

To describe the technique a number of definitions must be given. The *hazard* at any specified time is the risk of death within a very short interval for an individual who is known to have survived up to that time. As might be expected the two concepts, hazard and *survival probability* are related, although the relationship is a rather complex one which need not be described here. Suffice to say that one can be determined from the other. The idea of hazard has quite a long history, being first used in studies of population mortality where it is referred to as the age-specific death rate. When the hazard is constant for all times the implication is that the risk of death is independent of the length of time an individual may happen to have survived. Thus a patient who has survived for three months has the same risk of immediate death as one who has survived for ten years. Although this might seem counterintuitive, the assumption of constant hazard has been used with some success in a number of survival studies. An alternative assumption might be that hazard increases with increasing survival time, which is roughly analogous to aging. A more realistic approach is to avoid making any specific assumption about the constancy or otherwise of the hazard and to allow it to be estimated from the data. This is the approach which was first used by Cox (1972) in his original paper.

The relative hazard for a patient with a particular combination of prognostic variable values at a specified time is the hazard for that combination of variables at that time, divided by the hazard at that time for a hypothetical patient whose prognostic variable values are all zero. This divisor is known as the baseline hazard and is merely a technical device—there is no implication that such a patient must exist.

For technical reasons it is mathematically more convenient to work in terms of the logarithm of the relative hazard, and Cox postulated that for any combination of prognostic variable values the log of the relative hazard can be written as a weighted sum of these values.[24] In the breast cancer example the weighted sum would involve three constants, the weights for age, size, and aggressiveness, and the weighted sum for a particular patient would be calculated by multiplying her age, the size of the tumour, and the measurement of its aggressiveness by the corresponding weights and summing the resulting values. The aim of the technique is twofold: firstly, to determine the values of the weights, and secondly to determine the baseline hazard. Once this has been accomplished a survival curve can be determined for any combination of values of the prognostic variables. If necessary a transformation may be applied to any of the prognostic variables if this will improve matters, for example by reducing the variability of the observed values.

To provide a concrete illustration of the method, consider the classical set of data analysed by Fiegl and Zelen (1965) in one of the first papers in this field.[25] For one group of 17 myelogenous leukaemia patients survival times and the corresponding white blood cell counts (WBC) are given in table 9.7. Since the white blood cell values are so widely dispersed, ranging from 750 to 100 000 a log transformation is used to reduce the variability so that the final results are not dominated by the largest values.

A plot of survival time against the logarithm of white blood cell count is shown in fig 9.7, and this suggests that it may be possible to use log WBC as a predictor of survival time.

When the data are analysed with the NANOSTAT package the value of the weight for log WBC is found to be 1·42 and when this is combined with an estimate of the baseline hazard, survival curves corresponding to selected values of the white blood cell

116

TABLE 9.7
Survival times and white blood cell counts for 17 patients with myelogenous leukaemia

White blood cell count	Survival times (weeks)	White blood cell count	Survival time (weeks)
2300	65	7000	143
750	156	9400	56
4300	100	32000	26
2600	134	35000	22
6000	16	100000	1
10500	108	100000	1
10000	121	52000	5
17000	4	100000	65
5400	39		

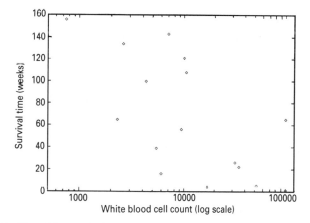

Figure 9.7   Plot of the survival times against white blood cell count based on the data given in table 9.7.

count can be calculated. Examples of white blood cell counts of 3000, 30 000, and 100 000 are displayed in fig 9.8. Thus the apparently rather vague indication of a relation between white blood cell count and survival time shown in fig 9.7 can be turned into a precise indication of survival.

However, like all exploratory statistical methods the proportional hazards regression technique must be used with a lot of caution and an adequate background knowledge of statistical

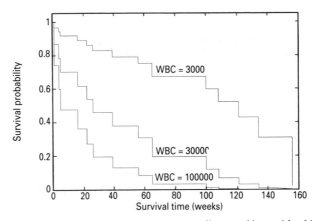

Figure 9.8 The estimated survival curves corresponding to subjects with white blood cell counts of 3000, 30 000, and 100 000.

science. It is easy to be misled when the data contains values which are particularly influential and so a full sensitivity analysis of the results is essential. The best advice is to enlist the help of a statistical expert when contemplating the use of this technique.

10
Sample size and power

Studies of the quality of statistical methods used in articles published in well known medical journals highlight the fact that many investigators pay insufficient attention to assessing what constitutes an adequate sample size for their study. A common error is to make the sample size too small or to fix on a number such as 20 or 50 for no other reason than it is a convenient round number, without any analysis of whether this will provide sufficient information to resolve the questions being asked.

Sample size determination ought to figure much more prominently in the planning of an investigation than it does at present. There is a simple reason for this: the primary aim of any comparative investigation is either to detect medically worthwhile differences between groups, or to demonstrate "beyond reasonable doubt" that there is no medically worthwhile difference between groups. Statistical analysis of data arising from a study which has used inadequate sample sizes will normally fail to detect all but the most extreme differences, so that small or moderate differences between groups which are nevertheless clinically important will usually pass undetected.

Early in the planning of a comparative study the investigator must address the following issues:

(a) What is the smallest medically important difference that the study should have a good chance of detecting?
(b) How large is the variability, measured by the standard deviation of the potential results, that is likely to be encountered?

Only by careful consideration of these issues can you arrive at a rational choice of sample size. Note the deliberate use of the phrase "a good chance of detecting" which is necessary because, when dealing with inherently variable measurements, you cannot be one hundred per cent certain of detecting a difference of a specified size.

119

		Actual situation	
		The population mean haemoglobin concentrations are the same for men and women	The population mean haemoglobin concentrations are not the same for men and women
The study data lead to the conclusion	No evidence of a difference	True negative result	False negative result
	Evidence of a difference	False positive result	True positive result

Figure 10.1   The possible combinations of actual situations and conclusions which could arise in a significance test for comparing population mean haemoglobin concentration in men and women.

An investigation that is too small is not only wasteful of resources but could be unethical in its use of patients in a situation where the investigation cannot achieve its stated aims.[26]

Significance tests and power

To understand the role that sample size plays in determining whether an investigation can achieve its aim it will be useful to continue the discussion of the example first introduced in chapter 3. This related to a study of haemoglobin concentration in men and women, the question of interest being whether the *population means* for men and women were different.

A significance test proceeds by setting up two opposing possibilities: either there is no difference between the population means or there is a difference. Analysis of the results of the investigation must then lead to one of two conclusions: either the data will provide evidence of a difference or they will fail to do so. The complexities of the situation are described in fig 10.1.

In the context of the haemoglobin study a false positive result would occur if the population mean haemoglobin values for men and women were equal but the study produced data that indicated they were different. Similarly, a false negative result would occur if the population mean haemoglobin values for men and women were different but the study produced data which suggested that they were equal.

The actual investigation compared measurements of haemoglobin concentration in the blood of 80 healthy men and a similar group of 80 healthy women. The sample mean (standard deviation) were 154·8 g/l (24·9 g/l) for men and 140·2 g/l (28·1 g/l) for the women. The difference between the sample means was therefore 14·6 g/l, and this was so large that it was regarded as providing very strong evidence to support the claim that the population mean haemoglobin concentrations for men and women are different.

The appropriate test is the two sample t test, and chapter 3 explained that the basic concept of the *sampling distribution* of the difference between the sample means played a fundamental part in establishing some of the properties of the significance test. Firstly, a single investigation will yield one value selected at random from the sampling distribution—in this example it would be the difference between the sample mean haemoglobin levels for men and women. Secondly, the sampling distribution has a mean that is equal to the difference between the population mean haemoglobin levels for men and women. Thirdly, the standard deviation of the sampling distribution is proportional to the population standard deviation of haemoglobin measurements divided by the square root of the sample size.

Figure 10.2(a) shows a hypothetical sampling distribution of the difference between sample mean haemoglobin concentrations when the underlying population mean concentrations are the same for men and women. This distribution is centred at zero and small or moderate differences are more likely to be encountered than large ones. The vertical lines are positioned so that they cut off in total the most extreme five per cent of the distribution. The standard convention is to treat a result which falls into either of these extreme tails as evidence of a difference between the population means, and consequently the difference of 14·6, which is very far out in the upper tail of the sampling distribution, is very strong evidence of such a difference.

A test which operates on this principle, that is treating as evidence in favour of a difference between the population means any observed difference between the sample means which is beyond either of the 5 per cent cut off points of the sampling distribution, has a P value of 0·05 or is said to be a test operating at the 5 per cent significance level. What this means is that if there is

121

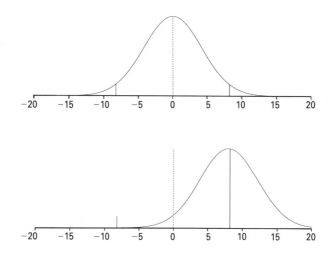

Figure 10.2   Sampling distributions of the difference between mean haemoglobin concentrations in 80 men and 80 women (a) when there is no difference between the population means for men and women, (b) when there is a difference of 8 g/l.

no difference between the population means, then the probability of getting a false positive result under this procedure is 5 per cent or one chance in 20. By operating this procedure we are assured that the probability of a false positive result cannot be more than 5 per cent. Of course there is nothing sacrosanct about the choice of 5 per cent, you could just as easily choose 1 per cent or 0·1 per cent, which would result in the cut off points being further out into the tails of the sampling distribution, just as you would expect.

Unfortunately, the choice of cut off points, which makes the probability of a false positive result small, automatically determines the probability of a false negative result. This would occur if there really is a difference between the population means but the difference between the sample means happens to fall somewhere between the cut off points. This is illustrated in fig 10.2(b) which shows the sampling distribution corresponding to a difference of 8 g/l between the population means for men and women. This sampling distribution is centred at 8 g/l and the probability of getting a false negative result is about 1 in 2 (50 per cent). The consequence of guarding against a false positive result, by requiring the difference between the sample means to be outside the cut

122

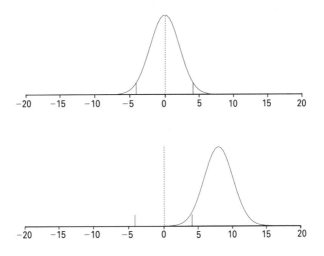

Figure 10.3   Sampling distributions of the difference between mean haemoglobin concentrations for men and women (a) when there is no difference between the population means for men and women, (b) when there is a difference of 8 g/l between the population means for men and women. The sample size is 320 in each group.

off points before it is accepted as evidence of a difference between population means, is that the chance of a false negative result is about 1 in 2 when the real difference between the population means is 8 g/l.

This apparent dilemma, that in setting a low chance of a false positive result we are automatically being forced to accept a high chance of a false negative result, can be resolved by using the fact that the standard deviation of the sampling distribution is proportional to the population standard deviation divided by the square root of the sample size. Increasing the sample size will decrease sampling distribution's standard deviation, for example a fourfold increase in sample size will halve the standard deviation. This is illustrated in fig 10.3, which shows the sampling distribution corresponding to samples of 320 in each group. Note the consequent reduction in the values defining the 5 per cent cut off point, which means that smaller differences between sample means qualify as evidence of a difference between the population means. Moreover, as fig 10.3(b) shows, the chance of a false negative result when the true difference between the population means is 8 g/l is greatly reduced, from about 1 in 2 when the sample size is 80 to about 1 in 20 with a sample size of 320.

To summarise, you may guard against false positive results by setting an appropriate P value (significance level) for the test, and by choosing the sample size carefully you may at the same time guard against a false negative result. The P value of the test is the probability of getting a false positive result, but the probability of getting a false negative result does not have a short name, although statisticians often denote it by the Greek letter β, so "beta value" might be one way of referring to it. The probability of getting a true positive result which is the chance that a difference that is real is actually detected is known as the *power* of the test.

The statements "there is no difference" and "there is a difference" are not of the same type: "no difference" means precisely that, but "a difference" covers a multitude of possibilities. For example, in the haemoglobin study the statement "there is a difference between mean haemoglobin levels in men and women" could refer to a difference of 0·1 g/l, 1 g/l, 10 g/l, or any other value. While the statement "there is no difference" is completely specific, the statement "there is a difference" requires further qualification before it is complete. This has important implications for the idea of the power of a test. You cannot refer to *the* power of a test as if there were one single number corresponding to a particular sample size, but must refer instead to the power of the test to detect a difference of a specified magnitude. This is illustrated in fig 10.4 which uses the data obtained in the study to graph the power of detecting differences of up to 20 g/l. Small differences have only a relatively small chance of being detected—for instance the test has at best a 20 per cent or 1 in 5 chance of detecting a difference of 5 g/l; but as the size of the difference increases, its chance of being detected also rises so that a difference of 20 g/l is virtually certain to be detected.

A test with a smaller sample size would have lower power throughout the range of potential differences, and this is illustrated in fig 10.5 which compares the power of the test based on groups of 80 men and 80 women with that based on 40 people in each group. The effect of increasing the sample size is quite appreciable in some parts of the range of differences but not in others. For example, a difference of 10 g/l has a chance of about 4 in 10 of being detected in the smaller study but is increased to about 7 in 10 by doubling the sample size; however, a difference of 5 g/l has only about a 1 in 10 chance of being detected in the smaller study and

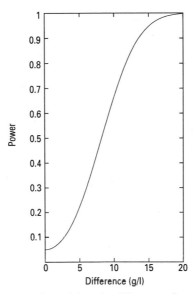

Figure 10.4   Graph of the power of detecting differences of up to 20 g/l between population mean haemoglobin concentrations for men and women for sample of size 80 in each group.

this rises to about 1 in 5 in the larger study. If the investigator needed to detect a difference of 5 g/l neither sample size would be adequate.

If power could be determined only after the study was complete then it would be an interesting but only partially useful concept. While it is useful to know after you have completed a study how powerful it was in detecting various sizes of difference, it would be much more useful to choose the power of the test in advance. The link between power and sample size makes this possible. All that the investigator has to do is to decide beforehand on the smallest difference that he or she wishes to detect and the power that the test should have of detecting that difference. In addition the investigator must have some information about the likely size of the population standard deviation, either from reports of previous studies or from a pilot study.

The Statgraphics package contains procedures which calculate sample sizes for certain standard tests and one of these, the "Sample Size—Normal Means" procedure can be used as a

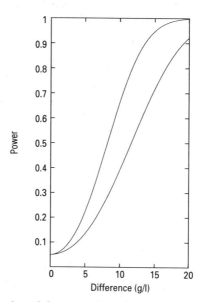

Figure 10.5   Comparison of the power of tests based on samples of size 80 (upper curve) and samples of size 40 (lower curve).

planning tool for investigations where the one or two sample t test would be used to analyse the results. Although the procedure is ostensibly designed to provide sample size for the single sample t test, minor modifications to the input data which the user provides enable it to be used for the two sample t test, and also for investigations involving the comparison of two proportions such as those described in chapter 7.

The input screen is shown in fig 10.6: the user is presented with a table rather like fig 10.1, except that it uses statistical jargon such as "type I error" to describe what we have called a false positive result and "type II error" to describe a false negative result. It also uses "HO" to refer to the situation where it is assumed that the population means are equal and "HA" to indicate that the population means differ.

Suppose that you wish to calculate sample sizes for the haemoglobin study which would enable you to detect a difference of 7 g/l or more between haemoglobin concentrations in men and women when the P value (false positive probability) is 5 per cent and the β value (false negative probability) is 10 per cent, assuming that the

126

Sample size—Normal means
True state of nature

	HO 0	HA 7
Decision		
Reject HO	Type I error Alpha = ·0500	Correct decision
Accept HO	Correct decision	Type II error Beta = ·1000

Assumed sigma = 35·4   Alt. hyp.: NE

Fixed sample size test
  Number of observations = 269
  Critical values for rejecting HO = − 4·23251 4·23251

Figure 10.6   The input and results panel for the Statgraphics normal means procedure.

standard deviation of the haemoglobin concentration measurements is 25 g/l for both men and women. This is done by keying in the values in the appropriate data input fields as shown in fig 10.6. You enter the values 0 and 7 in the fields immediately below the symbols "HO" and "HA," the *P* value of 5 per cent is entered as the decimal value ·05 in the field labelled "Alpha = " and the beta value of 10 per cent is entered as a decimal value ·10 in the "Beta = " field. In order to use the procedure to calculate sample sizes for a two group comparison the value which must be entered in the field labelled "Assumed sigma = " is not the assumed population standard deviation (remember the statisticians use the Greek letter σ to denote a population standard deviation), but the assumed population standard deviation times the square root of two, which in this case means that the value to be entered is 1·414 times 25 g/l or 35·4 g/l. The data entry is now complete and a few seconds after the procedure begins to run it produces the appropriate sample size which is 269.

A similar modification is used to induce the procedure to calculate sample sizes for comparing two population proportions. For example, the data in table 7.1 indicate that the proportion of healthy individuals with the Km 1 immunoglobulin allotype is about 55 per cent in healthy Indonesian subjects. Suppose that you wished to have a 90 per cent chance of detecting a reduction to 40 per cent or less in the pulmonary tuberculosis patients, how large would the sample size have to be if you proposed to set the *P* value of the test at 5 per cent? The completed data panel is shown in fig

Sample size—Normal means
True state of nature

Decision	HO 0	HA 0·15
Reject HO	Type I error Alpha = ·0500	Correct decision
Accept HO	Correct decision	Type II error Beta = ·1000

Assumed sigma = 0·706   Alt. hyp.: GT

Fixed sample size test
  Number of observations = 190
  Critical values for rejecting HO = 0·084311

Figure 10.7   The input and results panel for the Statgraphics normal means procedure when used to determine sample sizes for testing a difference between two proportions.

10.7. There are two points to note: firstly, the value entered for the assumed population standard deviation is calculated from the formula

$$\text{Assumed population standard deviation} = \sqrt{(2 \times p \times (1-p))}$$

where p is the average of the proportions of the Km 1 allotype assumed for the control and the patient populations, so that in this case $p = (0·55 + 0·40)/2 = 0·475$, so that the value to be entered is $\sqrt{(2 \times 0·475 \times 0·525)}$ or 0·706. The procedure produces the value 190 as the sample size for each group.

Formulae for calculating approximate sample sizes are so simple that you do not need a computer package to do the calculations. The formula for calculating an approximate sample size, denoted by n, for two equal groups for a two sample t test is

$$n = \frac{2\sigma^2(z_p + z_\beta)^2}{d^2}$$

where σ is the assumed population standard deviation, d is the smallest difference one wishes to detect, and some typical values of z_p and z_β are given in table 10.1.

By substituting the appropriate values into this formulae we find that the sample size for the previous example is

TABLE 10.1
Critical values for sample size determination.

		P value of the test	
	P = 10%	*P* = 5%	*P* = 1%
z_p	1·645	1·96	2·576

		False negative probability		
	β = 20%	β = 10%	β = 5%	β = 1%
z_β	0·845	1·282	1·645	2·326

$$\frac{2 \times 25^2 \times (1·96 + 1·282)^2}{7^2}$$ or 268, which agrees well with the value given by Statgraphics.

A very similar formula provides approximate sample sizes for comparing two population proportions, provided neither proportion is expected to be close to either zero or one. The required formula is

$$n = \frac{(z_p + z_\beta)^2}{2d^2}, \text{ where } d = \arcsin \sqrt{p_1} - \arcsin \sqrt{p_2}.$$

Applying this formula to the Km 1 immunoglobulin allotype study and substituting the appropriate values we find the sample size required for a test with a *P* value of 5 per cent, which is capable of detecting a reduction of 15 per cent or more in the patient population proportion when the control population proportion is 55 per cent is $\frac{(1·645 + 1·282)^2}{2 \times 0·1508^2}$ or 189, which is once again quite close to the value given by Statgraphics.

As a further aid to sample size determination Altman published a simple chart which allows you to read off approximate sample sizes for comparing population means or population proportions.[27][28] The determination of sample sizes for a wide variety of situations is the subject of two recent books.[29][30]

As the reader should now appreciate, the basic ideas are simple and all that is required to make a rational choice of sample size is some preliminary work to decide on (a) the size of difference one wishes to detect, (b) the risk of getting a false negative result that one is prepared to accept, and (c) a reasonable approximation to the numerical value of the population standard deviation. Providing this last value is admittedly difficult but there can be few situations where no information whatsoever is available. If it is the case that you are working in a totally new area where there is no information about variability, then obviously a pilot study will be an essential first step, since without the information that it will provide it is difficult to see how any rational planning can be carried out. Apart from its value in providing vital information for sample size calculations a pilot study allows you to try out the logistics of the investigation, and eliminate any flaws before they have a chance to render the investigation ineffective.

11

Writing up statistical analysis in a scientific paper

No matter how proficient a researcher may be at statistical analysis the final results are only as good as the data on which they are based. This means that the design of a study is of supreme importance. Take time to plan carefully before moving on to the collection of data. A carefully formulated investigation with a clear set of questions which are capable of being answered in an unambiguous manner is the objective. At the planning stage decide on what are likely to be adequate sample sizes using the ideas outlined in chapter 10. This means that you should have a clear idea of how the data are going to be analysed even at the planning stage. Never embark on an investigation where data are collected without anyone being sure of how they will be analysed, since more often than not this will result in a flawed study which turns out to be virtually impossible to analyse in any meaningful way. An incorrect analysis of high quality data can almost always be put right with a relatively small amount of effort, but a basic flaw in the design of a study means that the resources committed to it have been wasted.

At the planning stage the following questions need to be asked:

- What are the objectives of the study?
- How can these be formulated as questions which may be answered by collecting the right kind of data?
- What type of data will be needed?
- How much data will be needed?
- What is already known about the variability that will be encountered?
- How will the data be analysed?

- Is there someone who can provide statistical advice if it is needed?

When writing up an account of work done describe clearly the objective of the study and the design used. The statistical analysis should be described with sufficient detail that in principle anyone with access to the data would be able to reproduce exactly the analyses which are reported. This does not mean that standard methods should be described in detail but they should be adequately referenced. Only methods that are new or are likely to be unfamiliar should be reported in detail. Papers in medical journals often show disparity between the description of investigative techniques, which frequently go into great detail, even giving sources for particular reagents, and the often cursory description of the statistical techniques, such as "t tests were used throughout and a P value of 0·05 was taken as indicating statistical significance," when an examination of the content of the paper makes it clear that much more was involved.

When it comes to the reporting of results the rule should be that sensible graphs are to be preferred to tables wherever this is practicable, showing as much of the data as possible so that the reader can judge the reasonableness of any conclusions. Summaries of measured data should indicate variability as well as location, and sample sizes should be clearly specified. Wherever possible main results should be reported as confidence intervals rather than as bare P values. Also, beware of multiple testing on the same data and avoid the practice of "data dredging" to find a few "significant" results. Keep in mind the original aims of the investigation and beware of opportunistic sifting through data of dubious quality with the hope of "something turning up."

A number of medical journals use statistical referees and it is worthwhile subjecting the account of a study to the kind of checklist such as a referee is certain to employ.

This book has presented several standard techniques of statistical analysis and has sought to emphasise the importance of using statistical analysis to answer the *right* questions. It will be apparent from the discussion of the misuse of correlation and regression techniques in the comparison of laboratory methods, and the discussion on the evaluation of diagnostic tests, that it is sometimes easy to lose sight of the questions central to a scientist's investigations in the search for a convenient statistical technique. The

Design checklist

- Have the objectives of the study been clearly and sufficiently described?
- Has the design of the study been clearly and sufficiently described?
- Is the design appropriate to the objectives of the study?
- Has the source of subjects used in the study been clearly described?
- Have the criteria for inclusion or exclusion of subjects been clearly set out?
- Is the sample of subjects used in the study relevant to the population to which the results refer?
- Was the size of the study based on statistical power calculations?
- Is the design acceptable?

Statistical analysis

- Are the statistical methods adequately described and referenced?
- Are the statistical methods appropriate?
- Is there evidence that they have been used correctly?
- Is the presentation of statistical data, in the form of tables, graphs, numerical summaries satisfactory?
- Are the main comparisons or results presented in the form of confidence intervals?
- Have the statistical analyses been correctly interpreted so that the conclusions drawn from them are justified?

investigator should always remember that it is stupid to use the wrong technique to answer an irrelevant question. By using the checklist above it will be possible to ensure that the investigation is well designed and the statistical analysis is relevant.

Finally, you should attempt to clear your mind of the idea that all that is important is the calculation of some result (any result) which has a P value small enough to allow the result to be declared "significant." At the risk of boring the reader we will reiterate our view that statistical significance should always be related to clinical or biological importance, and a full measure of commonsense (with clinical or scientific insight) should be exercised in planning an investigation and interpreting the results.

12
Common statistical packages

Over the past few years the development of the Windows environment for personal computers has meant the look and feel of many statistical packages has tended to converge. Almost all packages now use menus to make selections rather than relying on commands, although many still allow the user the short cut of using commands to avoid having to make a series of selections from different menus to accomplish a particular task.

Minitab

The latest version of Minitab allows the user to select analyses and statistical methods from pop-up menus as well as by typing commands. This has the virtue of providing an easy way into the package for first time or occasional users, while allowing the experienced user to progress more rapidly. There is an excellent on-line help system which provides the user with useful information on such things as the exact syntax of commands and the various analyses that are available in the subsections of the package. There is a comprehensive user manual and a published book *The Minitab Handbook* which is both a guide to the major features of Minitab and a statistical textbook, although it is oriented to the general non-medical user of statistical methods.

The package does not contain methods for survival analysis but Minitab commands may be strung together as what are known as "macros," which allow the user to construct analyses that are not part of the standard package. A collection of macros comes with the package, and among these there are procedures for performing survival analyses.

There is a Minitab Users' Group and a regular newsletter is published by Minitab which contains news, features, and listings of macros that users have contributed. For academic users with access to e-mail (via the Joint Academic Network or JANet in the UK) there is now an e-mail discussion list. This sends out useful information about the package and allows users to send in questions and comments by e-mail.

The package is available in the UK from:
CleCom Ltd., The Research Park, 97 Vincent Drive, Birmingham B15 2SQ.

Statgraphics

Statgraphics has always been menu based making it easy to use by the first time or occasional user. All Statgraphics commands may also be invoked by typing short mnemonic commands, for example "REG" to perform a simple regression analysis. There is an excellent on-line help system which is accessible within any procedure; this provides context-sensitive help, giving details of the input required to make any procedure work correctly. There is a very comprehensive user manual running to over 800 pages, containing a wealth of useful information and examples of how to use each procedure.

As its name suggests one of the important features of the package is its extensive use of graphics both on-screen and in hard copy form. The package supports a wide range of graphics devices and it is easy to produce customised graphics displays.

The package contains all the usual univariate analyses plus a selection of multivariate analyses for handling certain aspects of multi-response data such as discriminant analysis. There is also a useful section which performs power calculations that enable the user to determine the minimum sample sizes needed to achieve statistical significance for a restricted range of common situations.

Available in the UK from:
Mercia Software Ltd., Aston Science Park, Love Lane, Birmingham B7 4BJ.

SPSS-PC+

SPSS-PC+ is a very extensive package that is able to perform analyses of an extremely wide range of single response and multi-response data. By virtue of its size it tends to be rather difficult for the first time or the occasional user, although there is now a Windows version of the package. There is a context-sensitive help system which can be called up to provide help on particular features and an explanation of terms which the user may find unfamiliar. The documentation is very extensive and comprehensive, including a number of published books at various levels. SPSS stands for "Statistical Package for the Social Sciences" so the tutorial documentation tends to treat examples of a non-medical nature.

The full SPSS system is relatively expensive and tends to use up quite a lot of hard disk space. This is probably a package more suited to the expert user who has large data sets to analyse rather than the occasional user with relatively modest requirements.

Available in the UK from:
SPSS UK Ltd., SPSS House, London Street, Chertsey, Surrey KT16 8AP.

SAS

SAS is another very large general purpose package. Extremely powerful and comprehensive in its coverage of statistical methods, virtually every analysis can be done in SAS. Its extreme power and complexity tells against it for the occasional user, since the system uses a command structure in which statements written in the SAS language control the processing and analysis of data. The user has to become familiar with the rudiments of this language before being able to do anything worthwhile. This of course means that it is not a package for those who need to perform analyses only at infrequent intervals since the learning curve is too long and the user will tend to forget how to do things.

The documentation is naturally very extensive with such a large package; stacked up there is about a metre of it. The most useful document is the *Introductory Guide for Elementary Statistical Analysis*. This contains a basic outline of statistical concepts as well as a step by step guide to the use of the base SAS software and the SAS/STAT software. The system is designed to comprise two basic steps—firstly, a DATA step where data are organised into an

SAS data set, then a series of PROC steps where the data is analysed using one or more of the SAS procedures. Each DATA and PROC step consists of SAS statements which have to follow the rules of the system: hence the difficulty for the novice or occasional user.

SAS is relatively expensive, but like SPSS it would be of greatest value to institutional users with a requirement for extensive analysis of large and complex data sets. It has become the standard package for statistical analysis throughout much of the pharmaceutical industry and so contains a wide range of procedures for the analysis of medically related data.

Available in the UK from:
SAS Software Ltd., Wittington House, Henley Road, Marlow SL7 2EB.

NANOSTAT

NANOSTAT is an easy to use package developed by Professor Michael Healy of the London School of Hygiene and Tropical Medicine. It is menu based. The menus are fairly utilitarian—the user is faced with a list of topics each indexed by a letter, together with the instruction to type the corresponding letter to invoke that section of the package. Once inside a section a similar menu allows a particular analysis to be selected with a further window-like screen to allow selection of the variables to be analysed, and so on. The occasional user should have no difficulty in working successfully with the package.

Graphical on-screen displays are available and there are some printer drivers for graphical hard copy, basically for the Epson, Hewlett Packard Laserjet, and Postscript ranges of printers.

There is on-screen help and a manual of about 140 pages. The system is reminiscent of Minitab and all of the standard univariate analyses are provided. One feature is the "More Statistics" part of the package, which contains a set of survival analysis methods and a number of other more specialised methods, such as logistic regression, principal components analysis, and canonical analysis. In addition this section contains the Wilcoxon and Mann-Whitney non-parametric tests.

This is a reasonably inexpensive package without any major shortcomings, and is of use to medical researchers with moderate requirements for data analysis.

Available in the UK from:
Alphabridge Ltd., 26 Downing Court, Grenville Street, London WC1N 1LX.

References

1 Pocock SJ. *Clinical trials: a practical approach.* New York: John Wiley and Sons, 1983.
2 Gore S, Altman DG. *Statistics in practice.* London: British Medical Association, 1982.
3 Armitage P. *Statistical methods in medical research.* Oxford: Blackwell Scientific Publications, 1971.
4 Bailey NTJ. *Statistical methods in biology.* London: Hodder and Stoughton, 1981.
5 Ingelfinger JA, Mosteller F, Thibodeau LA, Ware JH. *Biostatistics in clinical medicine.* 2nd ed. New York: Macmillan, 1987.
6 Diem K, Lentner C, eds. *Documenta Geigy, Scientific tables.* Basle: Geigy, 1970.
7 Gardner MJ, Altman DG. Confidence intervals rather than p values: estimation rather than hypothesis testing. *Br Med J* 1986;**292**:746–50.
8 Rothman K. A show of confidence. *N Engl J Med* 1978;**299**:1362–3.
9 Miller RG. *Simultaneous statistical inference.* New York: Springer-Verlag, 1981.
10 Conover WJ. *Practical non-parametric statistics.* New York: John Wiley and Sons, 1980.
11 Sprent P. *Quick statistics.* London: Penguin, 1981.
12 Neave HR. *Elementary statistics tables.* London: Allen and Unwin, 1981.
13 Kowalski CJ. On the effects of non-normality on the distribution of the sample product moment correlation coefficient. *Applied Statistics* 1972;**21**:1–12.
14 Gayen AK. The frequency distribution of the product moment correlation coefficient in samples of any size drawn from non-normal universes. *Biometrika* 1951;**38**:219–47.
15 Altman DG, Bland JM. Measurement in medicine: the analysis of method comparison studies. *Statistician* 1983;**32**:307–17.
16 Bland JM, Altman DG. Statistical methods for assessing agreement between two methods of clinical measurement. *Lancet* 1986;**i**:307–10.
17 International Standards Organisation. *Statistical tolerance intervals, ISO standards 3207.* Geneva:ISO, 1980.
18 Conover WJ. *Practical nonparametric statistics.* New York: John Wiley and Sons, 1980:111–6.
19 Griner PF, Mayewski RJ, Mushlin AI, Greenland P. Selection and interpretation of diagnostic tests and procedures: principles and applications. *Ann Intern Med* 1981;**94**:553–600.
20 Anonymous. When is a test diagnostic? [Editorial.] *Hum Pathol* 1985;**16**:325.
21 Prentice CRM, Forbes CD, Morrice S, McLaren AD. Calculation of predictive odds for possible carriers of haemophilia. *Thromb Diath Haem* 1975;**34**:740–7.
22 Fisher RA. The use of multiple measurements in taxonomic problems. *Ann Eugenics* 1936;**7**:179–88.
23 Morrison DF. *Multivariate statistical methods.* Tokyo: Kogakusha/McGraw-Hill: 1976:230–45.

REFERENCES

24 Cox DR. Regression models and life tables (with discussion). *J R Stat Soc [B]* 1972;**34**:187–220.
25 Feigl P, Zelen M. Estimation of exponential survival probabilities with concomitant information. *Biometrics*, 1965;**21**:826–38.
26 Altman DG. Misuse of statistics is unethical. In: Gore SM, Altman DG, eds. *Statistics in Practice*. London: British Medical Association, 1982:1–2.
27 Altman DG. How large a sample? In: Gore SM, Altman DG, eds. *Statistics in Practice*. London: British Medical Association, 1982:6–8.
28 Altman DG. *Practical statistics for medical research*. London: Chapman and Hall, 1991:455–60.
29 Desu MM, Raghavarao D. *Sample size methodology*. London: Academic Press, 1990.
30 Kraemer HC, Thiemann S. *How many subjects*. Newbury Park, California: Sage Publications, 1987.

Acknowledgements

We are grateful to the former editor of the *Journal of Clinical Pathology*, Professor G Slavin, for commissioning the articles which form chapters 1 to 8 of this book, to Mr R S Fawkes and Dr J H Gibbs for assistance in the preparation of the figures, to Miss M C K Browning of the Department of Biochemical Medicine, Ninewells Hospital and Medical School, for allowing us to use the data on TSH assays in chapter 6, and to Professor C D Forbes of the Department of Medicine, University of Dundee, for giving us access to the data used in chapter 8 on factor VIII concentrations in women who may be carriers of haemophilia.

Index